Behavior and Cancer

*Life-Style
and Psychosocial Factors
in the Initiation
and Progression of Cancer*

Sandra M. Levy

Behavior and Cancer

Jossey-Bass Publishers

San Francisco   •   London   •   1985

BEHAVIOR AND CANCER
Life-Style and Psychosocial Factors in the Initiation and Progression of Cancer
by Sandra M. Levy

Copyright © 1985 by: Jossey-Bass Inc., Publishers
433 California Street
San Francisco, California 94104
&
Jossey-Bass Limited
28 Banner Street
London EC1Y 8QE

Library of Congress Cataloging-in-Publication Data

Levy, Sandra M.
    Behavior and cancer.

    (The Jossey-Bass social and behavioral science series)
(The Jossey-Bass health series)
    Bibliography: p. 213
    Includes index.
    1. Cancer—Psychosomatic aspects. 2. Cancer—Social
aspects. 3. Life style. I. Title. II. Series.
III. Series: Jossey-Bass health series. [DNLM: 1.
Behavior. 2. Behavioral Medicine. 3. Life Style.
4. Neoplasms—etiology. 5. Neoplasms—psychology.
QZ 202 L668b]
RC 262.L44   1985   616.99'4071   85-45061
ISBN 0-87589-661-8

Manufactured in the United States of America

JACKET DESIGN BY WILLI BAUM

FIRST EDITION

Code 8537

A joint publication in
The Jossey-Bass
Social and Behavioral Science Series
and
The Jossey-Bass Health Series

Preface

Of all the afflictions to which the human body is subject, cancer is without doubt the most fearsome and mysterious. Its causes are only now beginning to emerge from shrouds of ignorance, superstition, and myth. Sontag (1978, pp. 60–61) remarks that cancer has been used metaphorically to express fantasies about strength and energy: "Whatever seemed ruthless, implacable, predatory could be analogized to cancer. . . . Cancer was never viewed other than as a scourge; it was, metaphorically, the barbarian within." Sontag wishes to uncouple personality, emotion, and behavior from organic disease, in order to place diseases such as tuberculosis and cancer in a proper, purely organic perspective. Her motives are humane, and her text is a brilliant commentary on modern medicine as it has emerged over the last two centuries from superstition and ignorance to objective science.

But despite her humane intention in letting illness be simply illness, without burdening the patient with additional fantasies, Sontag goes too far in her willingness to disengage psyche from soma. In recent years a number of writers (Miller, 1978; Ader, 1981; Herd, Weiss, and Fox, 1981; Schwartz, 1983) have developed a view of human health and disease from an integrative, systems perspective. And even before the emergence of such fields as behavioral medicine and health psychology, European writers such as Polanyi (1958) and Merleau-Ponty

(1962) conceived of human functioning in terms of an integrated structure, with human intention and behavior affecting somatic experience. Using other language, Ader (1981) concludes that a "purely" biological process, such as immune function, is fundamentally homoestatic and can finally be understood only in the context of the complex human or animal host interacting with its environment. Ultimately, he argues, this integrated, homeostatic set of mechanisms is under the control of the central nervous system. Therefore, higher cortical functions, via subcortical pathways, affect all levels of somatic functioning.

This volume is concerned with the relationship between human behavior and cancer. The linking pathways between human response and cancer development are numerous and complex, direct and indirect. There is, in fact, a current controversy over the amount of cancer risk to be attributed to the environment, and hence at least partly controllable by public health measures, and the amount to be attributed to "host factors," ranging from genetic predisposition and current health status to personal habits. Depending on one's point of view, then, one can emphasize either personal responsibility for lifestyle behaviors (such as smoking or excessive sunbathing without the use of sunscreens) or governmental, regulatory control over pollution and toxic contamination.

This controversy not only has an empirical basis, which will be closely examined throughout this book, but also, I suspect, philosophical and probably political and economic bases as well. A thorough analysis of these latter themes would require a separate text. But one should at least be aware of all the issues involved, as well as the probable multiple sources of opinion. The following excerpt provides a flavor of the "environmentalist" point of view. In a chapter entitled "What You can Do to Prevent Cancer," Epstein (1979, pp.465–466) states:

> It is perfectly true that we can make changes in our personal lives and habits that may significantly reduce our chances of getting cancer, but the possibilities are limited. An asbestos worker with

a growing family may well have a true grasp of the dangers he is exposed to, but in all probability he is firmly locked into his particular work situation. Modern industrial society offers most people little opportunity to choose freely where to live, where to work, what air to breathe or water to drink, what food to eat, and what advertisements to read or see. We must be willing to accept the fundamental reality that a *significant* reduction in exposure to environmental carcinogenics will result only from organized political action. The system of checks and balances leading to decision making must protect the overall interests and welfare of the public. This is the essence of democratic practice. Until very recently, congressional decisions and regulatory policy have too often reflected the overwhelming pressures and influences of industry without significant balance by consumer and labor interests.

On the other hand, writers with a personal responsibility perspective tend to emphasize individual choice and behavior in preventing disease. For example, Calabrese (1979) argues that the role of the environment in carcinogenesis is overestimated. He concludes that, although environmental factors may initiate and/or promote 85–90 percent of all cancers, this attribution of cause is misleading, since it neglects the critical role of the individual's health status as a factor modifying carcinogenesis.

No one would deny that some risk factors, such as smoking, are a matter of "life-style." It is also obvious that some of these personal factors interact with environmental sources of carcinogenesis—such as are found in the workplace. At the same time, the source of other risk factors lies totally outside the sphere of individual behavior—like being the recipient of an atomic bomb attack (although, even here, someone is "behaving" on the other end). Certainly, as Epstein (1979) points out, scientific data are not clear-cut and easily interpretable, and again multiple factors probably interact overall to contribute to various cancer risks. But although we may not be able to tease out here the amount contributed by environment and host, we know that ultimately both are important. In this book we will be primarily concerned with the behavior of individuals and groups, and with what can be modified at those levels of analysis.

Although a number of popular and scientific texts focus on selected aspects of this volume, there is currently no other comprehensive treatment of the role that behavior plays in the cause and progression of cancer. This work is aimed at a broad audience comprised of professionals and practitioners in psychology, sociology, health education, nursing, biology, and medicine, as well as advanced undergraduate and graduate students in these areas. Clearly, all readers can draw life-style implications for disease prevention and for early detection of disease where social and behavioral factors contribute to health risk. Certainly, those who are being trained for clinical practice—whether in psychology, nursing, or general medicine—will also benefit from intervention implications inherent in the topics covered.

During my years as chief of the Behavioral Medicine Branch at the National Cancer Institute, I gained a broad view of behavioral factors and cancer risk. I was also in a position to know the best of the research in this area. The National Cancer Institute also supplied the resources and support for the breast cancer project that is detailed in this volume (Chapter Seven). Therefore, this writing has a unique source and provides the most comprehensive coverage to date in the field of behavioral medicine and cancer.

This book was written in the hope that we can begin to untangle myth from reality and, in doing so, shed light on what can be changed to reduce cancer risk. Cancer is a complex disease, with multiple causes and contributors to outcome. Behavior is one of the factors in the equation. And behavior can be changed. All who read this book should derive not only knowledge of the role that behavior plays in cancer risk but also hope that, in light of this knowledge, such risk can be reduced. It is an enterprise worth all of the effort.

Plan for This Book

We are not concerned here with questions of mental health, psychopathology, or commonly understood psychosocial quality-of-life issues. That is, instead of viewing symptoms as mental health *sequelae* of disease (anxiety, distress, pain, and so forth), we will be viewing them as indirect or direct *contributors* to the disease process. We make no a priori assumptions about the psychological "healthiness" of response patterns but merely attempt to characterize behavioral patterns systematically as they seem to be associated with and potentially contribute to cancer incidence or survival. One could conceive of these independent, rather than dependent, variables as having an indirect or a direct effect on disease status. The accompanying table displays these

Relationship Between Behaviors as
"Independent Variables" and Cancer

	Direct Effect	*Indirect Effect*
	A	B
Initiation of Disease	Ultraviolet exposure	Sexual behavior
	Tobacco use	Fatty diet
	Alcohol consumption	
	Occupational carcinogens	
	C	D
Progression of Disease	Central nervous system effects on endocrine and immune function	Screening/detection behaviors and noncompliance
	"Stress"	
	Helplessness versus control	

potential associations. For example, behavioral noncompliance with optimal therapeutic regimens as a consequence of giving up or actively seeking alternative, unorthodox treatments would conceivably have an indirect effect on the course of the disease and treatment outcome (cell D). One would assume that opting for coffee enemas rather than surgery for early-stage colon cancer would not be associated with optimal treatment outcome. On the other hand, depression and behavioral helplessness are potentially mediated by sympathetic-adrenal-medullary release of catecholamine. Epinephrine, in turn, has been found to increase a type of immunological effector cell (T-suppressor cells), potentially suppressing immune control over micrometastasis (the early spread of relatively few malignant cells). This latter pathway is an example of a more direct effect of behavior on disease outcome (cell C).

As can be seen by a perusal of chapter headings, the topics can be placed within the matrix provided on the table. Chapter One provides a brief discussion of cancer epidemiology and tumor biology. This will give the reader a basic grasp of cancer as a disease process and will lay the foundation for all that is to follow. Chapters Two and Three address discretionary lifestyle factors associated with cancer risk. Specifically, Chapter Two considers factors such as sunlight exposure, alcohol and tobacco use, and occupational carcinogens and draws behavioral implications for reduction of disease risk. Chapter Three examines the evidence linking sexual behavior and diet to various forms of cancer and provides the reader with an evaluation of these much-publicized and emotionally laden topics. Chapter Four is concerned with indirect contributors to cancer progression (factors associated with delay in diagnosis, for example) and considers the evidence for the efficacy of various cancer-screening modalities, such as breast self-examination. This chapter also addresses the thorny issue of noncompliance with standard treatment and provides the practitioner with concrete suggestions for compliance enhancement strategies. Chapters Five and Six are primarily biological in content, addressing central nervous system–mediated effects on both tumor immunity and hormone regulation of tumor response. These two chapters were written by specialists in these fields, in order to provide the reader with an in-depth coverage of current knowledge in the areas of brain and immunity, as well as hormones and cancer. Chapter Seven reviews both animal and clinical research related to behavioral effects on cancer progression, and Chapter

Eight provides a summary of the evidence linking behavioral response and neoplasia, addressing both treatment and life-style applications.

Therefore, the scope of this work is a broad one. Our focus will be on behavior in its broadest sense as a biological response modifier relevant to cancer incidence and progression of disease. Deliberately excluded is a consideration of behavioral patterns and psychosocial sequelae of cancer—for example, a discussion of rehabilitation issues—because texts dealing with these topics are currently available. What is not available is what this book provides: a serious and critical examination of the role that behavior plays as contributor to the cancer process.

Acknowledgments

One of the most valuable contributors to this volume is Madelon Kellough, who appled her considerable typing and word processing skills to the preparation of this manuscript. She patiently labored through many hours of dictation in the process.

Substantive and stylistic review of the entire work was provided by my husband and colleague, Leon H. Levy. To him, and to my two sons, Brian and Kevin, I express my deepest gratitude for their patience and support for this enterprise.

Pittsburgh   SANDRA M. LEVY
September 1985

Contents

The Author

Sandra M. Levy is associate professor of psychiatry and medicine, and program director for behavioral medicine in oncology, at the University of Pittsburgh School of Medicine. Before joining the faculty at Pittsburgh, she was chief of the Behavioral Medicine Branch at the National Cancer Institute, Bethesda, Maryland. While at the National Cancer Institute, she held a faculty appointment in psychiatry at the Johns Hopkins University School of Medicine and a faculty appointment in oncology at Georgetown University School of Medicine. Levy was awarded the Ph.D. degree in clinical psychology from Indiana University, Bloomington, in 1975.

Levy's major interest over the last several years has been in examining the role that behavior plays as a biological response modifier relevant to cancer risk and progression. She has been particularly interested in studying aspects of the immune system and the effects of central nervous sytem input on various types of lymphocytes, relevant to tumor control or spread. More generally, as a behavioral scientist she has written extensively about behavior as it contributes to cancer control.

Levy has edited *Biological Mediators of Behavior and Disease: Neoplasia* (1982) and *Cancer, Nutrition, and Eating Behavior* (with T. Burish and B. Meyerowitz, 1985). She has also published numerous articles and chapters related to behavior and its role in the prevention and treatment of cancer. She is a consulting editor for the *Journal of Human Stress* and *Rehabilitation Psychology* and is an elected member of the Academy of Behavioral Medicine Research.

Behavior and Cancer

Life-Style
and Psychosocial Factors
in the Initiation
and Progression of Cancer

1

❈❈❈❈❈❈❈❈❈❈❈❈❈❈

Introduction: Relationship of Behavior and Cancer

There is no way of knowing exactly how many new cases of cancer occur each year, because in some parts of the United States cancer is still not a reportable disease. However, since 1973 the National Cancer Institute has gathered population-based incidence and survival data from eleven cancer registries, including tumor registries for Puerto Rico and Hawaii. These data, collectively referred to as the Surveillance, Epidemiology, and End Results Program (SEER), represent the most accurate estimate of cancer cases and survival in this country.

Table 1 displays incidence data broken down by major cancer sites. These data exclude "minor" cancers, such as carcinoma *in situ* (or noninvasive cancers) and nonmelanoma skin cancers. As can be seen, approximately 910,000 new cases of serious cancer were projected to be diagnosed during 1985 (American Cancer Society, 1985), as compared with a known incidence of 785,000 new cases of serious cancer in 1980.

Figures 1 and 2 reflect forty-eight-year mortality rates per hundred thousand population by sex. For females the most striking increase from the early 1950s to the late 1970s was in deaths

1

Behavior and Cancer

Table 1. Estimated New Cancer Cases by Sex for All Sites, 1985.

Site	Estimated New Cases		
	Both Sexes	Male	Female
All Sites	910,000[a]	455,000[a]	455,000[a]
Buccal Cavity & Pharynx (Oral)	28,900	19,500	9,400
Lip	4,500	4,000	500
Tongue	5,200	3,300	1,900
Mouth	10,400	6,100	4,300
Pharynx	8,800	6,100	2,700
Digestive Organs	215,200	109,500	105,700
Esophagus	9,400	6,600	2,800
Stomach	24,700	15,000	9,700
Small intestine	2,200	1,100	1,100
Large intestine ⎱ (colon-rectum)	96,000	44,000	52,000
Rectum ⎰	42,000	22,000	20,000
Liver & biliary passages	13,400	6,700	6,700
Pancreas	25,200	13,000	12,200
Other & unspecified digestive	2,300	1,100	1,200
Respiratory System	159,200	110,100	49,100
Larynx	11,500	9,500	2,000
Lung	144,000	98,000	46,000
Other & unspecified respiratory	3,700	2,600	1,100
Bone	2,000	1,100	900
Connective Tissue	5,000	2,700	2,300
Skin	22,000[b]	11,000[b]	11,000[b]
Breast	119,900[c]	900[c]	119,000[c]
Genital Organs	167,200	92,300	74,900
Cervix uteri	15,000[c]	–	15,000[c]
Corpus, endometrium (uterus)	37,000	–	37,000
Ovary	18,500	–	18,500
Other & unspecified genital, female	4,400	–	4,400
Prostate	86,000	86,000	–
Testis	5,000	5,000	–
Other & unspecified genital, male	1,300	1,300	–
Urinary Organs	59,700	41,500	18,200
Bladder	40,000	29,000	11,000
Kidney & other urinary	19,700	12,500	7,200
Eye	1,800	900	900
Brain & Central Nervous System	13,700	7,700	6,000
Endocrine Glands	11,700	3,500	8,200
Thyroid	10,600	2,900	7,700
Other endocrine	1,100	600	500

Table 1. Estimated New Cancer Cases by Sex for All Sites, 1985, "Cont'd."

| | Estimated New Cases | | |
Site	Both Sexes	Male	Female
Leukemias	24,600	13,600	11,000
Lymphocytic leukemia	11,800	6,700	5,100
Granulocytic leukemia	12,100	6,500	5,600
Monocytic leukemia	700	400	300
Other Blood & Lymph Tissues	43,300	22,400	20,900
Hodgkin's disease	6,900	3,900	3,000
Multiple myeloma	9,900	5,000	4,900
Other Lymphomas	26,500	13,500	13,000
All Other & Unspecified Sites	35,800	18,300	17,500

Note: Incidence estimates are based on rates from the National Cancer
Institute's SEER Program 1977-1981.

aCarcinoma in situ and nonmelanoma skin cancers not included in totals.
Carcinoma in situ of the uterine cervix accounts for over 45,000 new cases annually,
and carcinoma in situ of the female breast accounts for over 5,000 new cases annually. Nonmelanoma skin cancer accounts for over 400,000 new cases annually.
    bMelanoma only.
    cInvasive cancer only.
    Source: American Cancer Society, 1985, p. 8.

from lung cancer, accounting for 5 percent of age-adjusted cancer death rates in 1951-1953 and for 17.8 percent of cancer
death rates in 1976-1978, or an increase of 250 percent. This
increase is believed to be caused by a dramatic increase in
female smoking during the midpoint of this century. With an
overall drop in smoking rates in our current younger female
population, this trend may well reverse itself by the end of
this century.

The cancer mortality trend for males over approximately
the last fifty years also shows a dramatic increase in lung cancer
deaths, again attributable in large part to tobacco use patterns.
There has also been a slight increase in esophageal and kidney
cancers.

Overall, during the last thirty years, there has been a 29
percent increase in mortality rates for males, mostly due to lung
cancer; for females there has been an overall slight decrease in
deaths from cancer in general—despite the increase in lung
cancer mortality in this group.

Figure 1. Female Cancer Death Rates by Site,
United States, 1930–1978.

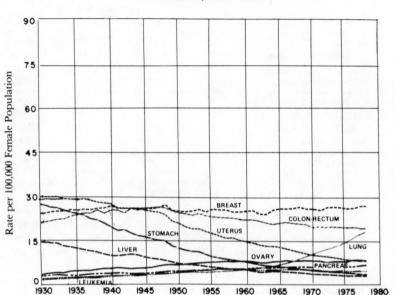

Year

Note: Rate for the female population standardized for age on the 1970
U.S. population.
  Sources: National Center for Health Statistics and Bureau of the Census,
United States.

The other side of the mortality data, of course, is the survival rate by cancer site. Five-year survival statistics from the
SEER program, for patients diagnosed between 1976 and 1981,
clearly indicate that patients with cancer are living longer than
ever before. The new statistics show that 50 percent of white
patients diagnosed with cancer during that period are curable
(or at least projected to be alive five years after the diagnosis).
When all races and sexes are combined, the figure is 49 percent, and this is a conservative estimate. It is also a preliminary
estimate, because complete five-year follow-up is available only
for patients diagnosed in 1978–79, and only for all cancer sites
combined. To the extent that the survival trend for patients will
improve as a result of improved treatment since 1980, these

Figure 2. Male Cancer Death Rates by Site,
United States, 1930–1978.

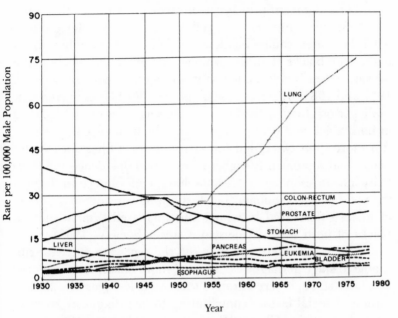

Year

Note: Rate for the male population standardized for age on the 1970 U.S. population.

Sources: National Center for Health Statistics and Bureau of the Census, United States.

figures may certainly underestimate the probability of five-year survival for patients diagnosed today.

Five-year relative survival (that is, the probability of escaping death from cancer for five years following diagnosis) is a fairly reliable indication of possible cure for most sites of cancer, excluding breast, prostate, and kidney. For patients diagnosed from 1950 to 1954 and followed by the National Cancer Institute for twenty years, 85 percent who lived for five years after diagnosis were still alive twenty years later. For sites such as breast cancer, this five-year survival as a sign of cure is less reliable because of the indolent natural history of this disease. That is, it is not uncommon for a woman to be disease free for ten years and then for the cancer to recur at a local or distant site.

Racial Differences in Incidence and Survival

The slight drop in survival rates when races other than white are taken into account reflects the fact that, for the past several decades, cancer incidence and mortality rates have been higher for blacks than for whites. For example, whereas the overall cancer incidence for whites was up 12 percent between 1947 and 1981, the rates rose 27 percent for blacks during that same period. Incidence of invasive cervical cancer has declined in both black and white females, but the incidence in blacks is still more than twice that found in whites. Other sites where blacks had significantly higher rates in both incidence and mortality include esophagus, prostate, lung, and colorectum. In fact, the incidence of esophageal cancer—long considered a disease of males—decreased in whites but increased dramatically in blacks of both sexes (American Cancer Society, 1985).

Survival differences between the races are partly attributable to stage at diagnosis. That is, more blacks are diagnosed at a later stage, where curative therapy is less feasible. Behavioral and social factors contributing to late diagnosis are considered in detail in Chapter Four. But according to a 1981 American Cancer Society–sponsored survey, urban black Americans as a group tend to be less knowledgeable than whites about cancer warning signals and less likely to see a physician if they experience cancer symptoms. They also tend to underestimate the prevalence of major cancers as well as the chances of cure from cancer in general.

Overall, then, incidence has remained relatively stable, with some fluctuations by site (for example, increase in lung cancer and decrease in stomach cancer incidence). Mortality has shown a decline over the last several decades, primarily because of combined, multimodal therapies and earlier detection techniques. Throughout this volume we will address behavioral factors that contribute to these incidence and survival figures, either directly (for example, by occupational exposure to carcinogens) or indirectly (for example, by diet or by treatment noncompliance).

Cancer as a Disease: Tumor Biology

Neoplastic (literally, new-growth) cells are broadly characterized as *benign* or *malignant*, although this distinction is sometimes histologically difficult to make, even for a sophisticated pathologist. The neoplastic growth is a persistently altered cell that reproduces itself, relatively uncontrolled by the animal or human host. "[In] the conversion of a normal cell into a tumor cell, a profound and heritable change occurs which allows the tumor cell to determine its own activities largely irrespective of the laws that govern so precisely the growth of all normal cells in an organism" (Braun, 1977, p. 46). This property of uncontrolled growth, referred to as *autonomy*, is the distinguishing characteristic of all neoplastic cells.

Benign and Malignant Tumors. Benign tumors typically do not spread throughout the body (that is, do not metastasize) and therefore tend to grow "in place." Such growths include common warts and moles and are usually quite harmless (although "benign" growths that develop in enclosed and vital spaces, such as the brain, are capable of killing the host by blocking essential vascular and neurological function). From a histological, or cell structural, point of view, the cells of benign tumors resemble the normal cells of the tissues from which they emerge and are classified according to their origin. For example, if such growths arose from bone, they are referred to as osteomas; from connective tissue, as fibromas; and so on.

Some features, such as autonomy, are general characteristics of both benign and malignant growth. But certain features of cellular structure and function belong solely to the malignant variety. In addition to the malignant tumor's ability to invade surrounding tissue and metastasize to distant parts of the body, microscopically the malignant cells are characterized by signs of *rapid growth* (multiple nuclei, multiple mitotic figures, indented and multiply shaped nuclei) and what is referred to by pathologists as *anaplasia*, or lack of form. Cells may appear haphazardly arranged, bearing little resemblance to the tissue from which they arose. When microscopic examination reveals that tumor cells have invaded blood vessels, normal tissues, or lymphatics, that is an unequivocal sign "that these cells are intrinsically dangerous. Death of the host will result unless these cells are removed or killed" (Pierce, Shikes, and Fink, 1978, p. 11).

As mentioned, the distinction between benign and malignant tumors is in many cases a matter of degree and is not always an easy one for the pathologist to make. The degree of surrounding tissue invasion (or stage of disease), the degree of anaplasia (or formlessness), and the rapidity of growth are all taken into account. Basically, clinical judgment must be made regarding how other similar tumors have developed under similar circumstances. Ultimately, "evidence of invasion or metastasis in the adult animal is diagnostic of malignancy" (Pierce, Shikes, and Fink, 1978, p. 13).

Categories of Malignant Tumors. The majority of malignant tumors in adults can be classified into two categories: sarcomas and carcinomas. Sarcomas arise from cells of connective tissue, such as tendons and bones; carcinomas arise from the epithelial cells that line the inner and outer surface of the body, such as those cells that comprise the skin or lining of the stomach. Malignant cells are also further classified according to their tissue of origin—for example, osteosarcomas, referring to malignant tumors developing from bone tissue. Carcinomas represent about 85 percent of all cancers in adults, and sarcomas represent approximately 2 percent. In addition, the incidence of carcinomas rises with chronological age. Therefore, as one grows older, one has a higher risk of developing breast or prostate cancer, for example. Incidence of sarcomas remains relatively stable across the lifespan. A twenty-year-old youth has approximately the same chance of developing bone cancer as a forty-year-old individual has.

Additional malignancies in humans are comprised of tumors that stem from immature blood cells, referred to as leukemias and lymphomas. Leukemia represents approximately 3.4 percent of all cancers in adults and is characterized by excessive white blood cells in the peripheral blood or bone marrow; lymphoma, a solid mass of immature white blood cells localized within the lymphatic system, represents approximately

5.4 percent of adult cancers. Again, the various subtypes of blood-derived cancers are categorized according to character and origin. For example, when the white blood cells that originate in the bone marrow become cancerous, myelocytic leukemia develops, with an enormous increase of leukemic, immature white blood cells in the peripheral blood. The balance of adult human cancers (about 4.2 percent) include tumors of the central nervous system and other malignancies that are not readily classifiable.

Case Examples of Benign and Malignant Tumors. The following two cases (from Pierce, Shikes, and Fink, 1978, p. 13) illustrate dramatically the biological differences between benign and malignant tumors. The hallmark characteristics of invasion and anaplasia of the malignant variety are illustrated in the second case.

> A fifty-two-year-old woman discovered a lump in her left breast, which proved to be rather tender and sore upon examination. She visited her physician, and, upon palpation, he noted that the lump was "rubbery" in texture and moved freely when examined. Palpation of her axillary lymph glands revealed no lymph node enlargement. Her physician performed a needle biopsy, and an examining pathologist found [that] the cells of the tumor . . . closely [resembled] normal breast tissue. He also found signs of a surface capsule which enclosed the tumor structure. He made a diagnosis of breast adenoma. The lump was removed and the patient pronounced cured. . . .

> A thirty-five-year-old female discovered a solid mass in her right breast, as well as some puckering of the skin over that breast area. She reported these symptoms to her physician, who found upon palpation a 3-centimeter, hard mass apparently fixed to the overlying skin and adjacent muscle tissue, suggesting tumor invasion of surrounding structures. Three hard nodules were also

found in her axillary lymph node region. A surgical biopsy was performed, and upon examination the pathologist found a highly anaplastic lesion, unencapsulated and infiltrating adjacent tissues. He also found fourteen of twenty lymph nodes examined to contain tumor cells. The majority of patients in such a diagnostic category develop widespread metastases, especially to the bone, liver, lungs, ovaries, and brain. This particular patient remained cancer free for thirteen months. She then developed a persistent cough and back pain. Tumors were identified in her lungs, liver, and pelvic joints. She was treated with both radiation and chemotherapy, but further tumors developed nine months later. She became emaciated and died. Although the cancer was by then widespread, the immediate cause of death was pneumonia. The cancer had sapped her body's ability to defend itself against infection.

Causes of Cancer

At the cellular level, according to Braun (1977) and others, it is a well-established fact that cancer can develop and exist in the presence of a completely normal complement of nuclear genes: "The basic cellular mechanisms that underlie the tumorous state are similar to those that underlie differentiation that occurs during the normal course of development in all higher organisms. Both phenomena depend for their expression on the persistent activation and repression of specific but, in part, different genes present in the nucleus of a cell" (Braun, 1977 p. 199). The questions currently at the forefront of scientific investigation concern the nature of genetic decontrol; the functions of oncogenes; and the mechanisms by which basic cellular processes are "switched" on and off inappropriately, triggering cellular disregulation and, ultimately, if uncontrolled, the host's death (Marx, 1984a). Recent research findings (Marx, 1984b) suggest that cancers of both nonviral and viral origins may be caused by the inappropriate activation of similar genes.

At a more macro level of analysis, the causes of cancer are multiple. In addition to understanding the genetic control of cellular expression, we also need to understand the triggering factors that affect this cellular behavior. In this book we are concerned primarily with understanding the links between the transformed cell and behavioral factors affecting cell and tumor behavior. In terms of *nature* and *nurture*, we are most concerned here with environmental and developmental nurture, because such factors can be at least partially modified. Certainly, nature cannot be ignored. As the British epidemiologists Doll and Peto (1981) point out, some individuals are born with genetic predisposition to certain cancers. For example, fair-skinned Caucasians are generally more susceptible to skin cancer than blacks. Women with first-degree relatives having bilateral, premenopausal breast cancer are at much greater risk for developing breast cancer than women not belonging to such cancer families. But not all fair-skinned individuals or all at-risk women get skin or breast cancer, even with the same exposure to environmental risk factors. So, in addition to an inherited tendency for developing certain forms of cancer, cellular abnormality on an individual basis is affected by individual-difference factors that may be more or less amenable to change.

Among the *nurture* factors that Doll and Peto (1981) list are environmental carcinogens (such as asbestos), endogenous and exogenous hormones (such as estrogen), obesity, reproductive history, "promiscuity," tobacco use, ultraviolet light, and viruses (such as hepatitis B virus). They do not consider "stress," which is potentially a modifier of host response (for example, immune surveillance), as a contributor to cancer risk. We will, however, consider the evidence in this area as well.

Concept of Host Vulnerability

According to Berg, Ross, and Latourette (1977), in their classic study of socioeconomic status differences in cancer survival, host differences associated with poverty can account for many of the black/white or poor versus advantaged survival differences. Such potential host differences include differential cell histopathology (for example, blacks more frequently exhibiting highly anaplastic tumors), immunological defect as a result of poor nutrition, and behavioral noncompliance with treatments. Clearly, some of these sources of host variance are more amenable to control than others.

Vulnerability stems from many sources and can be characterized in various ways. For example, there is a tumor/host vulnerability that is governed in large part by the histocompatibility characteristics of the host and the pathogen. In this regard Riley, Fitzmaurice, and Spackman (1982) note that selection of the proper tumor/host combination is critical in experimental animal model research. Both the perfectly compatible (syngeneic) and the histologically incompatible (allogeneic) models prove to be rather impervious to behavioral effects, the former because of minimal host resistance and the latter because of the elicitation of the host's immunological response, independent of behavioral influence. For our purposes here, particularly in regard to cancer progression, we are most concerned with slow-growing tumors, potentially under at least partial control of endogenous factors such as hormones or the immune system. The vulnerable host in this case—made vulnerable by behavioral, social, and life-style factors—is the concern of this volume.

2

✖✖✖✖✖✖✖✖✖✖✖✖✖✖✖

Direct Contributors to Cancer: Sun Exposure, Alcohol and Tobacco Use, and Occupational Hazards

Alfred Schutz (1899–1959), the Viennese philosopher and writer concerned with man's experience in society, characterizes the world of working as the fundamental reality of everyday life. In the translated collection of his writings (1973, pp. 226–227), he comments:

> The world of working as a whole stands out as paramount over and against the many other subuniverses of reality. It is the world of physical things, including my body; it is the realm of my locomotions and bodily operations; it offers resistances which require effort to overcome; it places tasks before me, permits me to carry through my plans, and enables me to succeed or to fail in my attempt to attain my purposes. By my working acts, I gear into the outer world, I change it; and these

changes, although provoked by my working, can
be experienced and tested both by myself and others,
as occurrences within the world independently of
my working acts in which they originated. I share
the world and its objects with others; with others
I have ends and means in common; I work with
them in manifold social acts and relationships,
checking with the others and checked by them. And
the world of working is a reality within which communication and the interplay of mutual motivation
become effective.

For Schutz play and other forms of social relaxation and
exchange take on "finite provinces of meaning," a shift in attitude and a suspension of the rules and order of the workplace.
This notion of work and play as fundamental aspects of living
that shape our perception of reality provides a backdrop for our
discussion of life-style factors and cancer risk. Because an individual's occupation has a central, organizing influence on his
or her life, the possibility that that same work environment might
harbor lethal consequences becomes all the more threatening.

The topics that we will consider in this chapter concerned
with lifestyle and cancer risk are intrinsically connected to work
or to social relaxation and play. If this intrinsic connection is
understood in a larger, fundamental human framework of living in a society that we shape and are shaped by, then we will
begin to understand why it is difficult to interrupt habits formed
by social intercourse and why individuals may continue to be
involved in socially formed work networks despite objective
danger.

In their epidemiological analysis of cancer causes, Doll
and Peto (1981) summarize the proportion of cancer deaths attributed to various factors (shown in Table 2). By far the largest
attributable estimates relate to tobacco and diet, together accounting for most cancer deaths. In fact, the only cause whose
effects are both reliably understood and numerically significant
is tobacco. Doll and Peto estimated that, in the United States
in 1981, tobacco would cause between 130,000 and 140,000

Table 2. Proportions of Cancer Deaths Attributed to
Various Different Factors.

Factor or Class of Factors	Percent of all Cancer Deaths	
	Best Estimate	Range of Acceptable Estimates
Tobacco	30	25–40
Alcohol	3	2–4
Diet	35	10–70
Food additives	< 1	– 5–2
Reproductive and sexual behavior	7	1–13
Occupation	4	2–8
Pollution	2	< 1–5
Industrial products	< 1	< 1–2
Medicines and medical procedures	1	0.5–3
Geophysical factors	3	2–4
Infection	10?	1–?
Unknown	?	?

Source: Doll and Peto, 1981, p. 1256.

deaths from cancer and that the percentage would continue to rise for a few more years, reaching about 33 percent of all cancer deaths by the mid 1980s. Allowing for some uncertainty in these estimates (because of possible misdiagnoses of lung and other types of cancers and because of the need to generalize from potentially atypical nonsmoking populations in order to estimate the small number of lung cancers not due to tobacco), Doll and Peto still insist that the current attributable risk for cancer death from tobacco use is somewhere between 25 percent and 40 percent. The American Cancer Society's (1985) figures also suggest that smoking accounted for about 30 percent of cancer deaths in 1985. Uncertainty regarding future risk is due to unknown, long-term effects of the current (and future) use of low-tar cigarettes.

As shown in Table 2, diet is the second most important modifiable source of cancer risk. Doll and Peto, citing evidence from animal and human research, conclude that dietary factors play an important, perhaps indirect or promotional, role in the development of cancers of the breast, endometrium, and gastrointestinal tract, although few firm conclusions can be drawn to date. We will consider this dietary evidence, as well as evidence concerning the effects of sexual behavior patterns, in detail in Chapter Three. This present chapter is concerned with life-style factors that play a potentially direct role in cancer incidence—namely, sunlight exposure, tobacco (along and synergistically interacting with alcohol consumption), and occupational carcinogens. In these two chapters, therefore, we address combined causal factors that potentially account for more than half (taking the mid-range estimate for diet) of all cancers.

Geophysical Factors: Ionizing Radiation and Ultraviolet Light

The following case (adapted from Krakowski, Tur, and Brenner, 1981, p. 271) illustrates the clear temporal connection between excessive sun exposure and the development of juvenile skin cancer.

> A three-year-old boy with red hair and a fair complexion was treated for a yellow-brown papule on his left shoulder. The papule had appeared when he was two years old. At the age of one year, after overexposure of his left shoulder to sunlight, he had a burn on this area. A vesicle appeared, which slowly faded, leaving a macule that changed to the papule.
>
> When the boy was four years old, a similar lesion appeared near the first one. During the next several months, the number of lesions scattered over the left shoulder gradually increased, and their color became reddish-brown. An ordinary black nevus, with two smaller ones near it, also appeared. A similar lesion was then noted on the right shoulder and another on the left abdomen. After about six months, the affected area on the left shoulder contained ten 5- to 9-millimeter lesions, five 2-millimeter lesions, and about forty lesions less than 1 millimeter in size.

During the next year, there was no change
in number or size, and the color faded somewhat.
The therapists avoided any intervention.

Unlike other forms of melanoma, juvenile melanoma is relatively "benign," and therefore treatment is usually conservative, as in the above case. For more aggressive forms of skin
cancer (squamous and basal cell carcinoma, as well as malignant melanoma), surgical resection is imperative.

Ionizing radiation and UV light were among the first factors recognized as cancer causing in human populations. UV
light is one of the principal causes of squamous and basal cell
carcinomas that occur mainly on the face, neck, and other
regions of the body exposed to the sun, particularly in fair-
skinned individuals. Melanoma, a more deadly sort of skin cancer, is rapidly rising in incidence among white-skinned populations and also correlates fairly highly with total amount of sun
exposure, worldwide. This worldwide increase in cases of melanoma may have come about because people now tend to wear
fewer clothes while engaging in outdoor work and play activity,
and hence are more exposed to UV light. However, this association with solar exposure is not as clear-cut in the case of melanoma as it is with basal and squamous cell carcinoma because
the distribution of affected body sites does not perfectly correspond to the amount of direct solar exposure to the sites. That
is, melanoma lesions are also increasing in bodily sites not directly exposed to UV light. One explanation for this increase
is that systemic hormones may stimulate melanocytes at distant sites. Doll and Peto (1981, pp. 1253–1254) attribute "90
percent of lip cancers and 50 percent or more of melanomas
as well as 80 percent of other skin cancer to UV light (lip cancer
in conjunction with smoking), in which case sunlight (especially,
strong sunlight on white skin) would account for between 1 [and]
2 percent of all cancer deaths."

A second geophysical factor that causes death from cancer
is ionizing radiation (the kind of radiation exposure that one
gets when one has a medical X ray or when nuclear "fallout"
occurs in the environmental vicinity). The relationship between

cancer incidence and this form of radiation is still subject to much debate and will not be discussed in this chapter to any great extent. Although there is still controversy over the dose-response relationship (for example, do dose-response effects differ from low-dose to high-dose exposure?) and over the amount of total or single-dose irradiation that is "safe" for practical purposes, it is assumed that "at low doses . . . the effect is approximately proportional to the dose" (Doll and Peto, 1981, p. 1254).

A pervasive source of ionizing radiation exposure in the United States is the medical use of radiation for diagnostic and treatment purposes. Such techniques are often essential for proper medical and dental care, and they probably account for 85 percent of the total ionizing radiation dose given in this country. Many of the recipients of radiation diagnosis and treatment are too old or infirm for increased cancer mortality in these populations to occur as a direct result of such exposure. That is, in all likelihood they will die of something else, most particularly the disease for which they are being treated. Although past use of medical radiation was less frequent, the dosage was higher than is currently given. Now the use of diagnostic and treatment radiation is more ubiquitous, but smaller dosages are used.

Considering the total use of radiation by medical practitioners—coupled with exposure to radioactive pollutants, to background cosmic rays, and to "the minute amounts of radon and other radionucleides that occur in the air, in our bodies, and in all natural materials and accumulate inside houses with restricted air exchange"—Doll and Peto (1981, p. 1254) estimate that the dose of radiation received by the population from background sources equals approximately 20 million rems per year, which would account for about 5,500 cancer deaths a year, or 1.4 percent of total cases. Together with an approximate 2 percent of cancer deaths caused by UV exposure, geophysical factors would then account for approximately 3 percent of all cancer deaths. They point out, however, that neither the background, "normal" environmental radiation nor sunlight can be entirely avoided. Therefore, cancer mortality risk that can actually be controlled—principally, the control of melanomas through avoidance of direct sunlight exposure in high-risk populations—is probably about 1–2 percent of total cancer mortality. For the balance of this discussion of geophysical factors, we will focus on UV exposure as, in part, a behaviorally controllable risk.

Ultraviolet Exposure and Skin Cancer. Skin cancers due to sunlight exposure are controllable only in part, because, although ultraviolet radiation (wavelengths between 250 and 320 nanometers, with 280–320 nm the most carcinogenic) is a causative agent in the development of many human skin cancers, certain racial groups (particularly those of Celtic origin) are more predisposed to skin cancer than other white population subgroups. Individuals with freckles, blue or gray eyes, little skin pigmentation, and light-colored hair are most predisposed to skin cancers of various forms. In contrast, Asians and blacks are significantly less prone to develop skin cancers. Allison and Wong (1967) noted that in Hawaii skin cancer is forty-five times less common in non-Caucasians than in Caucasians. Aging also increases the risk for developing skin cancer, and individuals with such genetic disorders as xeroderma pigmentosum (characterized by a reduced ability to repair solar-induced DNA damage) have a greatly increased risk for malignant skin lesions (Cleaver, 1978). Thus, although behavioral and environmental factors play a large role in the development of skin cancer, the host's susceptibility (due to genetic factors) and the chronological aging process itself, play a role in susceptibility. Although the focus here is on controllable exposure, these other sources of risk variance should not be forgotten.

Effects of Solar Radiation on the Skin. Strictly speaking, we are not concerned with the effects of "sunlight" here but with the adverse effects of exposure to the portion of the electromagnetic spectrum with wavelengths between 250 and 320 nm. These are ultraviolet wavelengths generated by the sun as well as by artificial sources. These ultraviolet wavelengths are not seen as light by the human eye, as are wavelengths greater than 400 nm. Infrared radiation, bands of wavelength above 700 nm, is experienced as heat. Wavelengths below 250nm are also very damaging to human skin, but fortunately the ozone-rich stratospheric layer of the earth's atmosphere absorbs these wavelengths.

What happens biochemically when the skin is exposed to significant UV radiation? Normal skin has several mechanisms that protect the organism from harmful exposure. First, visible light and infrared radiation are reflected to various degrees by white- and black-skinned individuals, but neither race can reflect the UV rays that are of concern here. Normal skin also absorbs a certain amount of such harmful energy, supplying a second natural protective mechanism during UV exposure. UV, infrared, and invisible radiation is absorbed by melanosomes within the epithelial layers of skin. Melanosomes are a first-line defense against solar radiation (Poh-Fitzpatrick, 1977). These reflective and absorbent defense mechanisms are bolstered by the phenomenon of scatter: "Subcellular organelles and macromolecular components of the epidermal cell . . . and intercellular optical discontinuities tend to deflect incident radiation from unimpeded direct transmission. As scattered radiation bounces about in the outer layers of the epidermis, its original energy is dissipated" (Poh-Fitzpatrick, 1977, p. 200).

Despite these defensive skin reactions, UV radiation still penetrates beyond the basal cell layer, lighter skin allowing more penetration than darker skin. One effect of such penetration is an increased number of melanosomes and a higher content of melanin within these cells. The result is either a deepened, overall shade of skin (a "tan") or an increase in number of physical "freckles" on the body's surface. As Poh-Fitzpatrick (1977) points out, when such tanning is understood as an attempt of the human body to shield itself from damage by UV radiation, the notion of a "healthy tan" becomes a contradiction in terms.

In addition to the acute effect of "sunburn" with which most of us are familiar (involving dermal vasodilation, increased vascular permeability, and various biochemical responses), UV radiation also can effect chronic, including malignant, changes in the skin. As a consequence of UV exposure, there follows an initial slowing of DNA, RNA, and protein synthesis, as well as a slowing of the process of mitosis, or cellular division. This depressed response is followed by an "explosion" of the same activities, apparently in an attempt to repair incurred damage.

This damage-repair cycle becomes accelerated through the repeated UV exposure. There is increased likelihood of both carcinogenesis and mutagenesis as a result of system failure or repair error related to this acceleration of a complex process (Poh-Fitzpatrick, 1977).

Although both basal and squamous cell carcinomas have been clearly linked with UV exposure, there is less evidence linking melanoma incidence with exposure to the UV portion of the solar spectrum. As indicated earlier, certain anomalies have shown up in the data, indicating that malignant melanoma is not as obviously associated with the most frequently exposed areas of the body; and reports of high incidence and mortality from melanoma in Scandinavian countries (Lancaster, 1956; Magnus, 1977) suggest that melanoma is not simply associated with more intense UV radiation exposure found near the equator. More recent epidemiological evidence sheds light on these anomalies.

Chrombie (1979) investigated the relationship between geographical latitude and melanoma incidence, using forty-three population-based cancer registries for both Europe and North America. He found that the North American and English melanoma incidence increased with decreasing latitude, suggesting an important causative role for UV radiation exposure. In distinct contrast, the incidence by latitude effect for Europe was in the opposite direction. That is, increasing incidence of melanoma was associated with increasing geographical latitude. Chrombie explained his findings by noting that across Europe there is a wide variation in skin color—from light in the Scandinavian countries to dark in the Mediterranean region. This range of pigmentation also provides an associated range of susceptibility to melanoma risk. ''The effect of this susceptibility must be large enough to overwhelm the opposing effect of decreased UV intensity at higher latitudes, and this emphasizes the danger of excessive solar exposure to fair-skinned individuals'' (Chrombie, 1979, p. 774).

For our purposes here, whether melanoma is a direct result of UV exposure or whether, as Blum (1978) suggests, sunlight is only an exacerbating factor in the development of mela-

noma, the exact causal mechanism of malignant transformation is less important than the fact that sunlight exposure plays
a major role in all forms of skin cancer, including its most
virulent variety.

   Animal Studies: The Search for Mechanisms. Most of the information on human skin cancer incidence derives from epidemiological data where only a small fraction of the population
studied is actually affected. Extrapolating to incidence as a function of increased UV dose requires that assumptions be made
about the nature of the dose-response relationship. These assumptions cannot be tested in human populations, so most of
the dose-response models or theories are based on animal data.
In a review of the animal photocarcinogenesis literature, Forbes
(1981) discusses various factors (such as the total dose of UV
delivered, the mode of UV delivery, and interactions with other
radiations or chemicals) that influence skin cancer susceptibility
in animals—principally hairless mice.

   There appears to be a dose-dependent response for tumor
development. That is, as the daily dose of UV exposure increases, an increased number of tumors develop in a shortened
period of time. But the situation is more complex than simply
amount of exposure. Forbes and his fellow investigators (Forbes,
1981) found that animals are more susceptible to tumors if they
receive the same total amount of UV exposure as comparison
animals but in smaller and more frequent doses. Specifically,
a weekly total dose was delivered on one, three, or five days
a week (smaller fractions of total dose given with increasing days
of exposure), for a total of forty weeks. Animals that received
a single, relatively large dose once a week had significantly longer
latent periods for tumor development that did animals receiving smaller doses three or five days a week.

   Forbes (1981, p. 139), drawing from these earlier laboratory findings, raised this issue of time-dose reciprocity related
to the potential long-term effects of occasional sunburn in human
populations: "Our limited experience with animal studies indicates that the influence of a relatively large dose 'pulse' is less
than what would be predicted on the basis of dose additivity
alone." That is, these data suggest that occasional bouts with

sunburn may have less of an overall, lifetime risk than more repeated, chronic exposure, although in smaller dosage. This may be especially true in Celtic populations and other groups at high risk for development of skin cancer.

In attempting to determine the exact carcinogenic wavelength action spectrum, Epstein (1978) noted that this determination has proved to be an almost impossible task to accomplish, because of the number of factors that need to be studied. For example, numerous potential wavelengths need to be assessed, both for their individual contribution and for potential interaction effects. In animal experimentation prolonged exposure periods, with large numbers of exposure intervals at each wavelength and at various intensities, are needed. Animals need to remain immobilized; and sophisticated, monochromatic source equipment, with minimal stray-light contamination, needs to be utilized. In addition to these complex "source" factors, between-strain differences in tumor susceptibility finally make a simple extrapolation to human risk problematic.

Animal studies have shown that the carcinogenic action spectrum in experimental animals ranges from 230 to 320 nm (Epstein, 1978). From available information the primary cancer-causing rays seem to be in the acute erythrogenic (sunburn) spectrum. Interaction with other wavelengths must also be considered. For example, longer UV waves (320–400 nm) significantly increase the acute damage caused by shorter waves: "Thus, . . . a determination of the action spectrum [and] a determination of the effects of various components of the sun's spectrum in cancer production comprise central subjects for further study" (Epstein, 1978, pp. 13–14).

Space does not permit further discussion of host and environmental factors that affect skin cancer incidence. Such factors as diet, animal strain, chemicals (for example, retinoic acids), heat, humidity, and wind have been shown to increase tumor production in UV-exposed animals. Since UV-exposed animals develop essentially no distinguishable basal cell carcinomas (a predominant form of human skin cancer) or melanomas, they have not provided a useful model for these tumor types. Animals do produce various epithelially derived tumors and can produce sarcomas under some conditions (Forbes, 1981). Therefore, generalization from experimental systems to the human condition must be done with care.

A final host factor that should be mentioned as a potentially important modulator of tumor response in UV-exposed animals is the immune system. Kripke and Fisher (1976, 1978), using a variety of techniques, demonstrated that chronically UV-irradiated mice do not reject highly antigenic UV-induced cancers, which are normally rejected by unirradiated, histologically compatible recipients. Their work suggests that UV irradiation specifically alters an animal's immunological responses to UV-induced cancers. These results, as well as other findings reported in the literature, suggest UV carcinogenesis enhancement following immunosuppressive changes (Forbes, Davies, and Urbach, 1979) and provide fairly convincing evidence that the host's immune system plays an important role in the development and control of skin cancer.

Prevention of Skin Cancer in Humans. In a somewhat acerbic conclusion to his review article, Forbes (1981, p. 141) expresses the following view: "If most of human skin cancer is caused by UV radiation exposure, then most such cancers are theoretically preventable . . . . In practice, it appears unlikely that most susceptible people will be convinced to abstain from UV radiation exposure, or to substitute skin painting for a sun-induced tan." Bennett and Robins (1977, p. 205) make the same point: "As with smoking and many another harmful activity, wanton disregard is still the common response. Sunbathing in frivolous pursuit of tanning goes on unabated." Since people evidently refuse to avoid needless exposure to sunshine, Bennett and Robins recommend the use of "topical preparations that mitigate the bad effects of the popular habit if properly chosen and used."

When we move from the realm of science to the realm of everyday human activity—which we will be doing throughout this book—we move from the realm of logic and facts (for the most part!) to the realm of human habit, preference, taste, and enjoyment within a social and cultural context. In order to change these habits and tastes, a massive campaign of health education may be required. Poh-Fitzpatrick (1977, p. 202) suggests that a "cultural revolution of sorts, with emphasis on the joys of sunrise swimming and twilight tennis, and acceptance of a fair complexion as beautiful" will be needed. Poh-Fitzpatrick also recommends a "propaganda" campaign for a daily application of a sunscreen as a regular grooming practice of high-risk individuals, beginning at a very young age.

In selecting a sunscreen for use, one should consider both the *protective factor* and the product's *substantivity*, as well as one's individual risk status. The protective factor is the ratio of the time required to develop erythema *with* a particular sunscreen to the time required for reddening without it. For example, a fair-skinned Caucasian will develop minimal redness in approximately a quarter of an hour of bright sunshine exposure. If a particular sunscreen allows such an individual to remain exposed to the same amount of sunshine for one and a half hours before "turning pink," that sunscreen's protective factor equals $1.5/.25 = 6$, a moderate degree of protection. Substantivity refers to the sunscreen's ability to resist washing off by swimming, perspiring, and so on.

Sunscreens primarily fall into two classes: chemical absorbers and physical reflectors of solar radiation. Some sunscreens allow tanning without burning; some allow neither. Some chemicals, such as menthyl anthranilate, absorb in both sunburn and tanning spectra; others, such as para-aminobenzoic acid (PABA), mainly absorb UV light in the sunburn spectrum. In advising physicians about counseling their high-risk patients regarding sunscreens, Bennett and Robins (1977) note that other factors, such as cosmetic acceptance, irritant potential, and cost, also must be considered. For example, products that reflect solar radiation and provide an excellent screen are generally opaque in quality and would be cosmetically unacceptable for general use.

The popularity of suntan salons for artificial tanning in this country and elsewhere is a reflection of the suntan cult and a testimony to how far public education needs to extend. As should be apparent from the content of this chapter, this practice has some cancer risk associated with it. Salons offer both

UVB (280–350 nm) and UVA (320–400 nm) light sources. The UVA wavelength is now viewed as more important in the tanning process than was previously assumed. Watson (1982) regards this shift in radiation source as fortunate, since many people will not only tan poorly with UVB radiation but will also add to their total solar damage by such potentailly carcinogenic UVB exposure. However, as he also notes, UVA exposure is not harmless. These longer wavelengths are partially responsible for aging effects, such as wrinkling, and there is evidence that UVA rays augment or potentiate skin cancer in animals who are also exposed to the shorter wavelength of UVB. Finally, large doses of UVA exposure (larger than for UVB) can cause sunburn of the skin. But in the absence of burn, it is difficult to control the dose received in UVA salons, so that "quite large doses can . . . be delivered without any discomfort to the patient" (Watson, 1982, p. 431). Kumakiri, Hashimoto, and Willis (1977) found that UVA exposure results in significant dose-related damage to several skin structures, including fibroblasts and nerve fibers. Watson (1982) concluded that, although UVA is more suitable for tanning than UVB, this artificial tanning method cannot possibly be endorsed as "safe" or without risk to skin and eyes. He also noted that the home use of such UVA equipment is particularly hazardous without the control of rigid safety standards.

In moderation, however, not all tanning is a bad thing— for those who can tan. Since sunlight is ubiquitous, some tanning provides a protective shield against its harmful effects. But prolonged, unnecessary exposure should be avoided; or, second best, the effects of such exposure should be minimized by the regular use of a suncreen agent. As a mostly Caucasian and therefore susceptible population, we cannot afford to wait until midnight swims, nighttime tennis, and pale skin become the preferred activities and mode.

Alcohol and Tobacco Use

The following fictitious case illustrates many of the risk factors associated with head and neck cancer. Poor nutrition, accompanied by chronic alcohol and tobacco use, is frequently part of the life-style history of individuals diagnosed with such malignancy. Overall prognosis is still relatively poor for such patients.

> Mr. Y., a fifty-five-year-old black male, presented at the outpatient emergency room of an inner-city hospital with complaints of a "lump" in his neck, as well as persistent hoarseness and weight loss. He had a twenty-year history of heavy smoking (two packs a day), combined with heavy alcohol consumption and obvious poor nutrition. Clinical and pathological examination revealed that the neck mass, along with neck nodes, was metastatic spread from a primary laryngeal malignant lesion. The primary laryngeal lesion was surgically removed, as were the mobile neck nodes. The remaining, inoperable nodes (inoperable due to tissue fixation) were treated with radiation. However, three months after primary treatment, recurrent nodes at the base of the skull became apparent. Despite further radiation visceral metastases developed, and Mr. Y. died seventeen months after the original diagnosis.

As Mr. Y.'s case demonstrates, alcohol and tobacco use frequently are found in the same samples of subjects, since people who smoke tend to drink. There is also evidence suggesting synergy between the two substances. Consequently, it seems desirable here to treat these two risk factors together.

Findings from a number of large-scale prospective studies (Rogot and Murray, 1980; Doll and Peto, 1976; Hammond, Garfinkel, and Seidman, 1977) clearly demonstrate the causal role of smoking in cancers of the lung, mouth, pharynx, esophagus, bladder, and probably pancreas and kidney. Smoking is thought to contribute to bladder and kidney cancer because tobacco smoke contains a variety of chemicals—some of which are mutagenic—that are absorbed into the blood through the lung apparatus and travel to distant bodily sites. These chemicals have been found in concentrated doses in smokers' urine.

Cigarette smoking produces the most widespread negative health effects of tobacco use, primarily affecting lung cancer incidence and mortality. These incidence and mortality rates are ten times greater in regular smokers than in those who have never smoked. Out of 71,000 lung cancer deaths observed in 1978, an estimated 64,567 (91 percent) were attributable to cigarette smoking (Doll and Peto, 1981). Cigarette smoking also plays a major role in the development of bladder and pancreas cancers. For cancers of the larynx, esophagus, mouth, and pharynx, all forms of tobacco use (pipe or cigar smoking, as well as cigarette smoking and tobacco chewing) are related to cancer risk.

Total Mortality Associated with Smoking and the Effects of Quitting. One method of estimating the total number of deaths attributable to smoking is to determine the male and female death rates from cancers of the lung, bladder, oral cavity, and so on, in a given time period and to compare the figure to the death rates that would have been expected if no one in this population had smoked. The resulting figure would be considered "excess" cancer deaths attributable to tobacco use. Taking this approach, Doll and Peto (1981) applied to the population as a whole the age-specific death rates of nonsmokers reported by the American Cancer Society (Garfinkel, 1980) for the period 1959–1972. Counting deaths from lung, bladder, pancreas, and upper digestive sites, they estimated an expected 40,000 cancer deaths in 1978 if no citizen had ever smoked. The actual mortality figure for those sites combined was 155,000, or approximately 115,000 excess deaths attributable to cigarette smoking.

Although this method is not perfect (for example, the original ACS sample may have been somewhat biased in terms of population characteristics, so that projection to the entire population based on these data may be faulty), other population predictions based on different data sets (Kahn, 1966; Doll and Peto, 1976) come very close to the ACS figures. Therefore, this projected figure of excess deaths attributable to tobacco smoking appears relatively accurate.

There is a dose-response relationship between cigarette consumption and cancer incidence, and this is a major reason for attributing causality to smoking for various cancer sites. Such a causal relationship is reflected in changing incidence as a function of number of years cigarettes are smoked, type of cigarettes used, depth of smoke inhalation, and age of smoking onset. This dose-response relationship is very strong for lung, oral, esophageal, and laryngeal cancers; the relationship is weaker for cancers of the pancreas, bladder, and kidney.

One implication of such a dose-response relationship between cigarette smoking and cancer is that when the behavior stops (the dose drops off), the risk of disease also decreases (the response subsides). This has been found to be the case for all of the tobacco-associated sites: ''The ex-smoker's risk of dying from lung cancer gradually decreases with the number of years off cigarettes and approaches that of the nonsmoker's after fifteen to twenty years, whereas for the continuing smoker the lung cancer risk [is] more than ten times that of the nonsmoker'' (Koop and Luoto, 1982). Likewise, the ex-smoker's risk for oral and laryngeal cancer decreases gradually and approaches risk for nonsmokers after ten to fifteen years. Risk drops off more rapidly for esophageal cancer, approaching the nonsmoker's risk after only four years of cessation. Koop and Luoto point out, however, that the person who has never smoked still has the lowest disease risk of all. The former smoker's residual risk for smoking-related disease effects is generally proportional to the lifetime exposure to tobacco smoke (Friedman, Petiti, Bawol, and Siegelaub, 1981).

As we saw in Chapter One, cancer death rates in the United States have continued to rise, with the percentage of predicted cancer deaths attributable to tobacco use increasing to about 33 percent in the mid 1980s. However, predicting trends to the end of this century is problematic because a number of unknown factors are involved in such an estimation. Increases in sales taxes, trends in public attitudes, development of ''safer'' forms of cigarettes, governmental regulations of various kinds, and so on—all will potentially contribute to risk and consequent mortality rates in decades to come. The accuracy of any prediction with such unknowns unaccounted for is clearly questionable.

Tobacco Chewing and Snuff Dipping. Chewing tobacco and

the use of snuff are becoming increasingly popular among adolescents. Snuff dipping refers to the practice of placing and re-
taining powdered or finely ground tobacco between the cheek
and gum. Winn and Associates (1981) investigated the relationship between snuff dipping and oral cancer in women in the
southeast portion of the United States, where snuff dipping has
traditionally been practiced. These investigators interviewed 255
women diagnosed with oral/pharyngeal cancer and 502 women
matched as a comparative control group. For the white women
in their case sample, the relative risk associated with snuff dipping among nonsmokers was 4.2. That is, women who used
snuff but did not smoke cigarettes still were four times more
likely to develop oral or pharyngeal cancer than women with
neither habit. Among chronic users of snuff, the risk approached
fiftyfold for cancers of the gum and buccal mucosa, tissues that
directly contact tobacco powder.

If the patients did not dip snuff, then the oral and pharyngeal cancers in this study appeared to be a result of the combined effects of cigarette smoking and alcohol use. Alcohol consumption was a risk factor in this study, but apparently only
among the women smokers: "When compared with persons who
had neither habit, there was a sixfold excess among persons who
were both heavy drinkers (equivalent to four ounces of whiskey
per day) and heavy smokers (two packs or more per day)" (Winn
and others, 1981, p. 748).

Although the incidence of cancer among snuff dippers is
lower than the incidence of smoking-related diseases, the increase
in production of smokeless tobacco over the last ten years (rep-
resenting a threefold increase in finely cut tobacco during this
time period), coupled with the heavy advertising campaigns
aimed at youth consumption, makes the results of this study
significant and ominous.

Passive Smoking. "Passive" or involuntary smoking, which
occurs when a nonsmoker is exposed to exhaled smoke or the
smoke of a smoldering product held between puffs, has been
implicated as carcinogenic in nonsmokers (Hirayama, 1981;
Trichopoulos, Kalandidi, Sparros, and MacMahon, 1981). Compounds found at higher concentration in sidestream smoke in-

clude ammonia and amines, nitrosamines, nitrogen oxides, and total particulate matter. However, these constituents also tend to be diluted in the air, and the particulates rapidly come to settle on nearby surfaces. As Koop and Luoto (1982, p. 323) have noted, "Many people find it [sidestream smoke] irritating; others who suffer from certain conditions such as heart disease or asthma find that it affects their health adversely. Children of smoking parents have been shown to suffer more bronchitis and pneumonia during the first year of life."

In 1981 three widely publicized investigations of the health consequences of passive smoking were published. Two of these, the Hiriyama and the Trichopoulos, Kalandidi, and Sparros reports, demonstrated a statistically significant increased risk of lung cancer among nonsmoking women of smoking husbands. The third study, reported by Garfinkel (1981), demonstrated an increased, but not a statistically significant, risk for nonsmoking wives. Although this evidence is limited by data and survey design, and does not allow firm, causative conclusions to be drawn at this time, Koop and Luoto (1982) have concluded that nonsmoker exposure to tobacco smoke should be limited as much as possible.

Studies of Mormons. A particularly interesting population subgroup that has been studied in recent years is the Mormons in Utah. Because of religious prescription and proscription, the Mormons on the whole are a relatively unique and self-contained group within which to study the effects of certain life-style behaviors on cancer risk. Doctrines of the Church of Jesus Christ of the Latter-Day Saints advocate abstention from tea, coffee, tobacco, and alcohol use, encourage large family size, discourage all extramarital sexual activity, and place heavy emphasis on education. And in fact, low cancer incidence has been observed in Mormons, especially in sites associated with alcohol and tobacco use, as well as in sites such as the rectum, cervix, breast, and ovary (Lyon, Gardner, and West, 1980).

In two recent studies, Gardner and Lyon (1982a, 1982b) stratified both male and female Mormons by degree of adherence to church tenets and then examined the causes of death in their sample. The males were divided according to their lay priesthood office, reflecting degree of adherence to church doctrines. Females were classified by degree of active church affiliation into inactive, possibly active, active, and very active categories. When thus stratifying by degrees of devoutness, these researchers did in fact discover that the most adherent church members of both sexes had significantly lower death rates for lung cancer than less devout Mormons did. Females active in church affairs had lower rates of cervical cancer; and devout males had lower rates of stomach cancer, leukemia, lymphoma, and other smoking- and tobacco-related cancers, such as esophageal cancer, than less adherent members did.

However, because other sites where differences had potentially shown up between Mormons and non-Mormons did not appear to be associated with adherence to church rules, Gardner and Lyon suggested that other characteristics and habits of this population might represent significant health-protective factors, unrelated to church rule adherence. For example, cancers of the breast and ovary are less frequent in Mormon than in non-Mormon women, but rates did not differ within the Mormon subpopulation as a function of church rule adherence. West, Lyon, and Gardner (1980) found little difference in number of pregnancies between active and inactive Mormon women but found large differences between Mormon and non-Mormon women in this regard. Therefore, whether or not one adheres to all the rules, church-associated life-style tendencies, such as preference for large families, may play an important and protective role in disease risk in such cultural groups.

Alcohol Consumption and Cancer Risk. Alcohol consumption has long been suspected of being carcinogenic, since cancers of the larynx, mouth, pharynx, and esophagus are more common in males whose occupations encourage large consumption of alcohol (Doll and Peto, 1981). However, precise figures for the percentage of such cancers directly attributable to alcohol consumption are hard to obtain. For one thing, self-report on amount of consumption is notoriously unreliable (Room, 1979). Second, as mentioned earlier, alcohol consumption tends to be associated with other habits, such as smoking, so that any independent causal attribution is problematic.

The totality of evidence indicates that, in the United States and Western Europe, the cancer-causing effect of even rather heavy alcohol consumption is fairly modest in nonsmokers, increasing the incidence of pharynx and oral cancer by two or three times (Rothman and Keller, 1972). In contrast, smokers who consume equal amounts of alcohol have a considerably higher risk for cancer of the larynx, esophagus, pharynx, and mouth. Doll and Peto (1981) attribute 3 percent of total cancer deaths in both sexes to alcohol consumption. They point out, however, that this attributable proportion cannot simply be added to that associated with tobacco use, since these two proportions largely overlap: "In other words, most of the 3 percent of cancer deaths now caused by alcohol could have been avoided by the absence of smoking, even if alcohol consumption remained unchanged" (Doll and Peto, 1981, p. 1225).

There has also been controversy regarding the differential risk of drinking spirits over other forms of alcohol consumption, such as wine or beer. Although Mashberg, Garfinkel, and Harris (1981) found that beer and wine drinkers have a much higher cancer risk than whiskey drinkers, the nature of their population studied—primarily individuals in lower socioeconomic groups—makes their interpretation of their findings problematic. Beer and wine are cheaper beverages to obtain—and therefore abuse. Moreover, other factors among the lower socioeconomic groups, such as poor nutrition and oral hygienic habits, could potentially enter into these findings. However, recent evidence suggests that one major effect is attributable to the alcohol itself, irrespective of its form. This conclusion has been underscored by the finding of increased rates of oral cancer among habitual users of concentrated, alcoholic mouth washes (Maclure and MacMahon, 1980).

Biological Mechanisms Underlying Host Risk in Alcohol and Tobacco Use. The mechanism of action related to alcohol-associated cancer risk is not understood, nor is the mechanism of interaction whereby tobacco and alcohol may jointly affect cancer risk (Koop and Luoto, 1982). Alcohol itself has not been demonstrated to be carcinogenic in animal studies. Perhaps alcohol facilitates the development of cancer by increasing the contact between carcinogenic agents (such as are found in tobacco products) and generative or stem cells that line the larynx and digestive tract.

Schottenfeld (1979) has proposed a number of biochemical and immunological mechanisms of action to account for the effects of alcohol as a "cofactor" in cancer causation. Among these mechanisms are immunosuppression and host susceptibility as a result of nutritional deficit. For example, both human and animal studies have shown that alcohol lowers leukocyte migration into damaged tissues to fight infection. But a direct causal relationship between alcohol consumption, immune suppression, and cancer risk is difficult to determine because malnutrition and other related host factors, such as liver disease associated with heavy alcohol consumption, cause suppression of cellular immunity. Berg, Ross, and Latourette (1977) attempted to account for excess cancer mortality in a sample of indigent patients by proposing that malnutrition and alcohol consumption contributed to host vulnerability. They speculated that the indigents may have experienced a "nutritionally caused difference in the implantation site 'soil.' There is a tendency for cancer cells to implant themselves where tissue is abnormal, and perhaps the connective tissue of the malnourished . . . is a favorable site for cancer [growth]" (p. 476).

Perhaps, then, alcohol-associated nutritional deficit—acting in association with other carcinogens, such as are found in tobacco products—increases host vulnerability to malignant change. Whether the association between alcohol and tobacco use is additive or synergistic, for our purposes here the fact of their joint contribution to cancer risk is of major importance.

Prevention of Smoking- and Alcohol-Related Cancers: Behavioral Implications. Both alcohol and tobacco use are part of the prevailing norms in Western society and hence are difficult if not impossible to eradicate. For example, it is obvious that individual drinking behavior does not exist in social isolation but is linked to the social character of reciprocity customs that surround it. If you serve me cocktails at your house, I feel compelled to offer you drinks when you come to mine. These habitual social activities may be so entrenched in our culture that "the prevention of oral cancer will prove difficult and . . . the decrease will more likely be controlled by early diagnosis" (Smith, 1979, p. 1196). Of course, some tobacco-related cancer sites, such as lung, are relatively incurable once discovered. That is, the concept of "early detection" is less relevant in these cases. Therefore, to reduce disease risk, tobacco appears to be the more important of the two substances to eliminate. Whereas moderation in alcohol use seems a reasonable position to assume, moderation in tobacco use is not.

Techniques used in the alteration of smoking behavior include self-help manuals, educational programs, clinics, drugs, hypnosis, behavior modification, aversive conditioning, and individual counseling. In general, outcome statistics have not been very encouraging. Most studies report only a 20–30 percent quit rate, at three- to six-month follow-up, irrespective of the approach used. These behavior change areas will not be reviewed in depth here. (See Leventhal and Cleary, 1980, for a review of this area.) Rather, the efficacy of the professional as change agent—particularly physicians but also others, such as dentists and nurses—will be considered.

There is a common lore that most people quit smoking on their own. Either they are finally convinced through heightened media awareness that smoking is personally harmful, or they become symptomatic and their physicians urge them to quit or face very adverse consequences—and they do stop tobacco use. The health professional as change agent is viewed as a powerful means to alter health-deleterious behavior. However, many smokers claim that they have never been advised by their physician or dentist to quit. In one survey (American Cancer Society, 1979), 70 percent of those smoking more than one pack of cigarettes a day said that they would quit if urged by their physicians to do so.

Lichtenstein and Danaher (1976) developed a model for various kinds of interventions that physicians can perform. These five roles include (1) acting as a healthy life-style model by not smoking; (2) providing information to patients about the risk of tobacco use and risk reduction if they quit; (3) encouraging abstinence by advice and suggestion; (4) referring patients to a professional smoking cessation program; and (5) prescribing use of specific cessation and maintenance strategies, and following up on outcome over an extended period of time. In a detailed and practical discussion of specifically what the physician (or other health professional) can do to facilitate smoking cessation, Sherin (1982) suggests the following strategies for intervention: encouraging the patient to set a specific quit date; helping the patient avoid triggers to smoke (such as coffee consumption or party attendance with other smokers); showing the patient how to manage weight gain by planning a specific change in diet; preparing the patient to anticipate unpleasant withdrawal symptoms—specifically, by training the patient in such techniques as systematic relaxation, meditation, or exercise; and setting up a "buddy system," where two patients who want to quit smoking may aid each other in the process. The health professional can verify the patient's self-report on follow-up visits by administering physiological examinations of smoking effects—that is, by measuring blood carboxyhemoglobin or saliva thiocyanate levels.

Actually, the role of physician as behavior change agent is not new. In the third decade of this century, Kress (1931) wrote of the physician's role in helping patients quit smoking. More recently Russell and his colleagues in England (Russell, Wilson, Taylor, and Baker, 1979), in a well-controlled trial using twenty-eight general practitioners, demonstrated the potentially important effect of physician advice. Intervention—consisting of two minutes of advice, a simple leaflet, and follow-up—produced a 5 percent one-year quit rate. If all general practitioners in the United Kingdom adopted this strategy, these researchers argue, there could be 500,000 ex-smokers a year.

It is interesting that the preponderance of follow-up studies of physician intervention have been done with general practice patients, pregnant women, or cardiac patients as target audiences. Typically, studies are not concerned with already diagnosed cancer patients. Upon reflection, this is not so surprising because, again, when the main smoking-related site (lung) is diagnosed as malignant, the probability of cure is so relatively low that smoking behavior becomes less relevant at that point. Clearly, the time to quit is before the cancer develops!

In general, the physician intervention outcome studies reveal two main trends: (1) Quit rates in more recent studies tend to be lower than in earlier work. (2) Rate of quitting goes up with severity of diagnosed disease. Pederson (1982) believes that recent quit rates are lower because more people are trying to quit on their own initiative; hence, only "hard-core" smokers—many with smoking-related diseases—find their way into physicians' offices. She also suggests that there may simply be more honesty in reporting, in part because of the availability of procedures for verifying self-reports (such as the use of the saliva thiocyanate test). Although such studies have attempted to isolate predictors of quitting success, many results are contradictory. For example, two studies (Mausner, Mausner, and Rial, 1967; Russell, Wilson, Taylor, and Baker, 1979) found that the initial amount smoked had an effect on quitting success, whereas two additional studies (Handel, 1973; Mausner, 1970) found no such effect. The most frequently supported relationship has been found with sex, males being more likely to quit successfully than females (Burns, 1969; Handel, 1973; Pederson, Williams, and Lefcoe, 1980).

Because of the scarcity of good research on the success of health providers in helping people stop smoking, only the most general conclusions can be drawn at this time. Certainly, follow-up monitoring of patient status should be carried out. Physiological measures of smoking effects for a verification of self-report should also be used, since at least one study (Sillett, Wilson, and Malcolm, 1978) showed that possibly 23 percent of those who reported abstinence actually were still smokers as defined by carboxyhemoglobin levels. Research carried out in this area has been relatively simple, investigators asking questions such as "Is there a differential quit rate associated with severity of diagnosed disease?" But studies of specific physician interventions in patient populations, systematically varying physician and patient characteristics (for example, physician communication pattern and patient health beliefs) and analyzed by multivariate technique, need to be pursued. The outcome of such research would allow physicians and other health service providers to predict which patients are likely to follow advice and to tailor their interventions for these patients in order to have the maximum effect.

Since, as mentioned, tobacco use—unlike sun exposure or alcohol—is unequivocally harmful at any dose, the best intervention obviously would be one directed at encouraging people not to take up smoking in the first place. (See Leventhal and Cleary, 1980, for a good review of the developmental process of tobacco addiction in its inception phase.) Some good beginnings have been made in this area, with specific intervention aimed at adolescents and even much younger children (Evans and others, 1978). In general, attempts have been made to educate youngsters about the immediate physiological effects of smoking, as well as long-term deleterious effects, and to "inoculate" them behaviorally so that they can resist peer pressures to take up smoking. The target behaviors are also beginning to be expanded to include tobacco chewing, because of the epidemiological evidence related to snuff dipping and oral cancer. Much of the media message related to this form of tobacco use is aimed at youth and enhances the attractiveness of chewing tobacco by pointing to adolescent folk heroes, such as baseball players, who engage in this activity.

Voluntary, discretionary behaviors such as these are generally under individual control. When we consider the question of individual versus societal responsibility for cancer risk reduction, however, perhaps we need to ask "What proportion of responsibility should be assumed by the individual and what proportion by society?" With the life-style factors we have been discussing, individual responsibility weighs heavily. In the next section, on cancer risk in the workplace, the larger proportion of responsibility may lie with governmental and industrial control of risk factors—although even here individual behavior is also very important. As Alfred Schutz and others (Berger and Luckman, 1966; Merleau-Ponty, 1962) eloquently describe, we finally live in a social matrix that supports our habitual, routine, and leisure behaviors. Perhaps we are our brother's keeper at all levels of involvement—from role model as parent to hostess providing party libations. If we live in a cancerogenic society, we as individuals must share the burden—for our own as well as others' behaviors.

Occupation and Cancer Risk

The following case, although fictitious, portrays a typical history of a worker exposed to probable carcinogens in the workplace, initiating malignant transformation of cells. Cancer (in this case lung cancer) appears clinically after years of subclinical growth.

Mr. F., a sixty-four-year-old white, was a construction worker who had worked at a naval shipyard during and after World War II, lining pipes and fittings with asbestos. He saw his family physician with complaints of a persistent cough, chest pains, and brownish phlegm, or rust-streaked sputum. Mr. F.'s physician had counselled him for ten years to stop smoking and had treated him for bronchial infections and persistent coughs before. However, the chest pains, sputum, and weight loss caused special concern, and his physician ordered chest films to be taken. Results showed the effects of bronchial obstruction and suspicious shadows suggesting regional metastases. Lung and bone marrow biopsy revealed that Mr. F. had small-cell anaplastic carcinoma; metastases were found in regional and abdominal lymph nodes and also in the pancreas. Because of the advanced nature of this lung cancer, Mr. F. was considered incurable. Therefore, only palliative radiation efforts were instituted to relieve his cough, bronchial obstruction, and pain. Mr. F. died four months after diagnosis.

Again, this is a typical case history, reflecting the probable cancer outcome following earlier exposure to asbestos in the line of work, coupled with chronic cigarette smoking, which interacts synergistically with the carcinogenic asbestos to contribute to subsequent cancer. By the time Mr. F. experienced reportable symptoms, the malignancy had widely metastasized, and the probability of cure was essentially nil.

Proportion of Cancer Incidence Attributable to Occupational Exposure. The first association between occupation and cancer risk was observed by a British surgeon, Percival Pott, in 1775. He reported a relatively high incidence of cancer of the scrotum—a generally rare disease—among chimney sweeps. In 1895 a German surgeon, Rehn, published his observations on bladder cancer in dye workers. Although this disease was uncommon in his day, Rehn diagnosed three cases of bladder cancer in a relatively brief period of time among workers in a small factory.

Occupational carcinogens continue to be recognized by clincial observation, both because of an extremely high ratio in exposed individuals, compared to the disease rarity in the population at large, and because of absolutely high incidence rates among exposed workers. However, the development of sophisticated epidemiological tools in more recent investigations has allowed the recognition of even moderately elevated risks (for example, a threefold risk), even for cancers that are not particularly rare in the population at large (Cole, 1977).

Table 3 shows established occupational causes of cancer. As a conservative estimate, Doll and Peto (1981) attribute an overall 4 percent of cancers in the United States to occupational exposure, with attributions of varying proportions for separate cancer sites (Table 4). Although 4 percent overall is a fairly small proportion of cancer deaths directly attributable to occupational exposure, it amounts to approximately 8,000 deaths in the United States every year. Occupational cancers also tend to occur within particular subgroups of workers (such as minority workers in the steel industry).

According to Doll and Peto (1981, p. 1245), occupational risks "can usually be reduced, or even eliminated, once they have been identified." That conclusion appears to be optimistic. Certainly, environmental carcinogens are a source of cancer risk that should be eminently controllable. However, there are complex issues involved in effecting such a reduction—issues that must be addressed through careful research. To date, they have gone unexamined.

Workers' Compliance with Protective Measures. A fundamental question for us to consider here is whether the individual

Table 3. Established Occupational Causes of Cancer.

Agent	Site of Cancer	Occupation
Aromatic amines (4-aminodiphenyl, benzidine, 2-naphthylamine)	Bladder	Dye manufacturers, rubber workers, coal gas manufacturers
Arsenic	Skin, lung	Copper and cobalt smelters, arsenical pesticide manufacturers, some gold miners
Asbestos	Lung, pleura, peritoneum (also probably stomach, large bowel, esophagus)	Asbestos miners, asbestos textile manufacturers, asbestos
Benzine	Marrow, especially erythroleukemia	Workers with glues and varnishes
Bischloromethyl ether	Lung	Makers of ion-exchange resins
Cadmium	Prostate	Cadmium workers
Chromium	Lung	Manufacturers of chromates from chrome ore, pigment manufacturers
Ionizing radiations	Lung	Uranium and some other miners
Ionizing radiations	Bone	Luminizers
Ionizing radiations	Marrow, all sites	Radiologists, radiographers
Isopropyl oil	Nasal sinuses	Isopropyl alcohol manufacturers
Mustard gas	Larynx, lung	Poison gas manufacturers
Nickel	Nasal sinuses, lung	Nickel refiners
Polycyclic hydrocarbons in soot, tar, oil	Skin, scrotum, lung	Coal gas manufacturers, roofers, asphalters, aluminum refiners, many groups selectively exposed to certain tars and oils
UV light	Skin	Farmers, seamen
Vinyl chloride	Liver (angiosarcoma)	PVC manufacturers
(not known)	Nasal sinuses	Hardwood furniture manufacturers
(not known)	Nasal sinuses	Leather workers

Source: Doll and Peto, 1981, p. 1238.

Table 4. Cancers That Definitely Can Be Produced by Occupational Hazards.

Type of Cancer	No. of Deaths Recorded in 1978		Cancer Deaths Ascribed to Occupational Hazards in 1978 (United States)			
			Male		Female	
	Male	Female	No. ascribed	% ascribed	No. ascribed	% ascribed
Mesentery and peritoneum	652	697	98	15	35	5
Liver and intrahepatic bile ducts	1,812	984	72	4	10	1
Larynx	2,909	550	58	2	6	1
Lung	71,006	24,080	10,651	15	1,204	5
Pleura, nasal sinuses, and remaining respiratory sites	857	496	214	25	25	5
Bone	997	740	40	4	7	1
Skin (other than melanoma)	1,061	753	106	10	15	2
Prostate	21,674	–	217	1	–	–
Bladder	6,771	3,078	677	10	154	5
Leukemia	8,683	6,708	868	10	335	5
Other and unspecified cancers	15,445	14,821	1,045	6.8	185	1.2
Subtotal, above sites	131,867	52,907	14,046	–	1,976	–

Source: Doll and Peto, 1981, p. 1244.

worker's behavior has any mitigating effect on carcinogenic exposure. If it does not, then there would be no reason for behavioral interventions of any sort, nor would there be any role for public health efforts aimed at individual or group response. However, there seems to be a range of controls in the workplace, extending from engineering devices to specific work practices. Where engineering controls are available, behaviors having to do with proper maintenance, responses to equipment failure, and so on, would be the most relevant to consider. On the other hand, specific protective work practices (such as the wearing of gloves or respirators (would be more important where engineering controls still allow workers to come into direct contact with hazardous substances. For example, in a 1978 special occupational hazard review of trichloroethylene (a commonly used cleaning solvent in many occupations and industries), the National Institute for Occupational Safety and Health concluded by stressing the importance of improved work practices. Among protective measures recommended were the use of protective clothing, institution of practices for cleanup of spills, establishment of good general housekeeping and sanitation practices (for example, avoiding food consumption in areas where TCE is handled), institution of practices for safe entry into confined spaces such as tanks, and long-term establishment of medical surveillance.

Related to various work practices, these behavioral procedures are typically developed by common sense and consensus. The practices themselves are rarely measured systematically (for example, quantifying the range of practice, with independent observers rating degree of perfection), nor, in most cases, are the specific practices validly correlated with actual exposure. But despite this lack of systematic behavioral measurement, we can still ask: Is there a problem in behavioral cooperation on the part of the worker? At least anecdotally, there is disagreement in this regard. Some report that there is no problem; management simply gives the protective equipment and then successfully educates the worker to use it. Others report that there is a real industry and worker compliance problem. Little "hard" data on actual plant and worker violations in exposure levels and recommended practices are available, but observations have been made of improper use of equipment and, in at least one instance, of total failure to utilize protective equipment in particular plants until "two or three days before we sent a hazard review team to their place. The workers told us that they never had used the equipment up until then" (National Institute for Occupational Safety and Health official, personal communication, 1982).

It is probably safe to assume that noncompliance rates differ by industry, plant size, socioeconomic status of the workers, and so on. It is virtually certain that there is a problem. We know from the general health promotion literature that people do not comply. For example, only a 40 percent compliance rate with long-term, prophylactic, health maintenance regimens has been reported in an extensive review of the compliance literature (Haynes, Taylor, and Sackett, 1979). However, we do not have systematic data on the extent of the problem—that is, the prevalence of noncooperation with optimal work practice—or on the extent of compliance with the work practices proposed. Nor are there data concerning the relationship between compliance with work practices and exposure reduction. These are basic research questions that should be addressed by systematic investigations in this area.

Because of these unknowns, behavioral implications to be drawn are less clear-cut in this area than in UV exposure or tobacco use. Of course, the latter risks—particularly smoking—are intrinsically contributive to occupational mortality. As Table 4 shows, cancers of the lung and other respiratory sites account for the largest percent of occupational cancer deaths in the United States. But even here, there is controversy over the proportion of cancer variance contributed by workers' smoking behavior and the amount contributed by other factors in the host and in the environment (Sterling, 1978).

Smoking and Workplace Cancer. Evidence has been produced concerning the potential interactive and mutually potentiating effect of smoking and workplace carcinogens, such as asbestos, in the production of various malignances. In a study of 370 asbestos insulation workers (Selikoff, Hammond, and Churg,

1968), the results showed that asbestos workers who smoked had eight times the cancer risk as smokers not exposed to asbestos. The legal implications of this finding are obvious, since many companies maintain that the workers' personal habit of smoking, and not environmental work exposure, produces cancer risk. In addition, as discussed earlier, the health implications of passive exposure to smoke have been extended to the work environment. In fact, legal suits have been filed by nonsmoking employees to force management provision of a smoke-free setting. In a suit settled in 1978, a Bell Telephone employee successfully sued her employer for the right to work in a smokeless environment. And in 1984 California voters passed an initiative forcing employers to provide smoke-free work areas if even one employee so desires.

In a review of the evidence on the contribution of tobacco use to workplace cancer, Mushinski and Stellman (1978) concluded that cancer of the lung is causally related to asbestos dust exposure in combination with tobacco smoke. In addition, available evidence suggests that tobacco smoke may act as a cocarcinogen with chromate, vinyl chloride, coke oven emissions, and chloromethyl ethers. And among individual carcinogens associated with bladder cancer are benzidine, beta-naphthlamine, and N-nitrosamine. Tobacco smoke contains certain of these amines, and therefore a strong interactive effect may be produced by exposure to both tobacco products and these various industrial chemicals.

Mushinski and Stellman also addressed the smoking habits of females in different occupational groupings and concluded that their risk for occupational cancer related to workplace and tobacco exposure will approach that of males when they are employed in similar industrial jobs. Stellman and Stellman (1981) hypothesize that stress in the workplace may play a motivating role related to female smoking patterns. Such stress arises in women workers because of pressure to perform a dual role of homemaker and wage earner. In addition, women tend to have less satisfying jobs and are paid less than male counterparts: ''When compared with men, women suffer from job discrimination, slow advancement, lower pay, and exclusion from decision-making processes. Many women smoke to relieve internal stress, whatever the source, and women as a group have a more difficult time quitting than men" (Stellman and Stellman, 1981, p. 30).

There are those, however, who view the whole issue of smoking as a health hazard in the workplace as a "smoke screen" to divert attention away from the effects of occupational and environmental exposures to toxic substances. In a provocative review of the research evidence, Sterling (1978) concludes that the relationship between smoking, occupation, and disease needs clarification. In fact, studies that have compared the smoking habits of groups of individuals "actually serve to contrast groups [that have] a high proportion of blue-collar workers exposed to toxic fumes and a low proportion of professionals, managers, and proprietors with groups having lower proportions of blue-collar workers and high proportions of professionals, managers, and proprietors" (Sterling, 1978, p. 437). Therefore, Sterling suggests, many diseases associated with smoking may actually be of work origin. At the least, the relative effects of smoking versus work exposure have yet to be determined. In addition to environmental contributions, host differences as a function of genetic susceptibility, as well as other intrinsic host factors, could certainly be playing a role (Calabrese, 1979).

Behavioral Implications for Workers. Even though the exact contribution of smoking to work-associated cancer is still uncertain, the overall importance of smoking cessation in general and the weight of the evidence indicating that smoking is a major contributor in some fashion to occupational cancer make it clear that the individual worker would decrease cancer risk by not engaging in this behavior. However, many aspects of the work setting—from stress to social support—play a role in maintaining this habit. For example, in many blue-collar occupations, the act of smoking is tied to social exchange in lounges and cafeterias. In fact, when smoking is not permitted in the immediate work environment, smoking breaks are typically provided. Some have suggested that workers in restricted areas may smoke more during breaks and after work to compensate for "lost" smoking during working hours. In addition, if smoking is limited to breaks, the positive quality of social interaction may reinforce tobacco use by pleasant association.

Although there have been a number of innovative smoking cessation programs in the industrial setting (educational campaigns, competitive teams with monetary bonuses as rewards for "winning," counseling, and so on), most programs have not been overwhelmingly successful, possibly because social reinforcement and stress reduction factors have not typically been taken into account in these efforts. Until we understand more completely the exact relationship between worker behaviors (specific work practices and specific job requirements in worker subpopulations) and varying disease risk within groups, little else can be scientifically recommended at this point except common sense, prudence, and observation of state-of-the-art exposure control as it is developed.

For most of the cancer sites affected by carcinogens, early detection by various screening techniques has not proved highly effective in reducing mortality. For example, the available data on screening for lung cancer have not yet shown that such screening has any value. Thus, "the implementation of large-scale screening programs for lung cancer . . . seems unwarranted, at least until more promising data appear" (McNeil and Eddy, 1982, p. 355). McNeil and Eddy do recommend screening for colon cancer in asbestos workers, since this population also has a relatively high risk of dying from this disease and the evidence suggests the cost-effectiveness of such a program for exposed workers. But in general, the impact of screening on cancer morbidity and mortality is uncertain, and at present many programs cannot be totally relied on (Cole, 1977, p. 1791).

Obviously, the prevention of occupationally associated cancers would be far better than early detection and treatment. Besides smoking cessation and prudent work practice, collective worker behavior in the form of unions and other lobbying bodies to promote a safer work environment is another possible course of action (Epstein, 1979).

Behavioral Implications for Health Care Professionals and Government. One of the most significant contributions that the clinician can make in aiding our understanding of occupational carcinogenesis and identifying risk factors to be controlled is in the careful recording of work history for every patient, particularly where cancer is suspected of being present. Cole (1977) suggests that such a work history can be helpful even if attention is directed only at the two jobs held longest. For each of these occupations, the health care provider should determine the individual's age, when the job started and stopped, and the specific work duties involved. This clinical investigation would maintain what Cole refers to as the "index of suspicion in what continues to be the front line for the identification of new cancer hazards in the work environment, the astute clinician" (p. 1791). The systematic pooling of such data from a large number of cases would enlighten us in regard to the incubation period (exposure duration and time since exposure) required for cancer to develop.

Doll and Peto (1981) also recommend collecting information on occupational exposure and linking it, for example, to a national death index. Despite heated political debates over occupational cancer, they point out, there is still no routine national system for generating reliable information related to occupational exposure and mortality. Milham's (1976) effort in the state of Washington to link certified cause of death with information about occupation that could be listed on death certificates was both inexpensive and effective in uncovering real workplace dangers. Such a system could be extended to other states. Cole (1977) and Doll and Peto (1981) also note, however, that, since most cancers take twenty years or so to develop, past agents discovered as carcinogenic now are no longer found in current work settings. Instead, other agents come rapidly into use whose cancer potential will not be known for many years.

The World of Work and Everyday Social Reality

We began this chapter with a quote from Alfred Schutz, where he describes the world of working as paramount. "I share the world and its objects with others; with others I have ends and means in common; I work with them in manifold social acts and relationships, checking with the others and checked by them. And the world of working is a reality within which communication and the interplay of mutual motivation become effective" (Schutz, 1973, p. 227). After examining the evidence and implications associated with sunlight exposure, tobacco and alcohol use, and occupational function, we need to draw back and reflect on the human import of what we have discussed.

It is not true that we are caught in a cancer epidemic, and it is not true that everything causes cancer. But some things do, albeit modified in their effect by host factors. According to Schutz and others, our world of primary significance is first and foremost a shared one. And to learn that where we meet—at work and at play—has potentially lethal aspects and consequences is profoundly disturbing. Because these same aspects are supported by culture and affect our whole sense of self and well-being, they are also difficult to modify.

3

✖✖✖✖✖✖✖✖✖✖✖✖✖

Indirect Contributors
to Cancer:
Sexual Behavior and Diet

The French phenomenologist Maurice Merleau-Ponty has noted
the profound significance of sexual behavior for humans:

> The importance we attach to the body and
> the contradictions of love are . . . related to a more
> general drama which arises from the metaphysical
> structure of my body, which is both an object for
> others and a subject for myself. The intensity of
> sexual pleasure would not be sufficient to explain
> the place occupied by sexuality in human life or,
> for example, the phenomenon of eroticism, if sex-
> ual experience were not, as it were, an opportunity
> vouchsafed to all and always available, of acquain-
> ting oneself with the human lot in its most general
> aspects of autonomy and dependence [Merleau-
> Ponty, 1962, p. 167].

Other writers using other language—from Saint Paul to Freud—
likewise bestow fundamental importance on human sexuality.

Similarly, the consumption of food and the sharing of the communal meal possess far greater significance then the mere sustenance of life. From the ancient writings of the Epicureans to Old Testament dietary strictures to Freud's characterization of oral fixation manifested in, for example, an oral dependent personality type, the manner of eating and the quality of that consumed represent, as well as create, basic definitions of the self in a social matrix.

Therefore, to consider risks for cancer associated with two aspects of the human condition that are fundamental to the definition of oneself—sexuality and food consumption—is indeed a disturbing prospect. In fact, once one grasps the basic human significance of these consumatory behaviors, then the near hysteria over, for example, possible dietary carcinogens or cancer risk associated with a homosexual life-style becomes more understandable. But the evidence—much of it epidemiologically and clinically derived—is there. What conclusions can be drawn from such evidence, however, remains problematic.

Sexual Behavior and Cancer Risk

The following case illustrates the potential cancer risk inherent in certain sexual life-style patterns:

> A thirty-five-year-old white man with a history of engaging in active receptive anal intercourse since his late teens was examined for rectal bleeding and was noted to have an ovoid, deeply ulcerative 2-cm-in-diameter lesion involving the interior midline of the anorectum at the level of the pectinate line. Examination of the biopsy material revealed an *in situ* and infiltrating cloacogenic carcinoma with transitional and squamous cell features [Cooper, Patchefsky, and Marks, 1979, p. 557].

Cloacogenic carcinoma of the anorectum, an uncommon form of cancer, arises from epithelial tissue identical in embryonic origin to tissue that forms the female uterine cervix. Women with squamous cell cervical carcinoma are known to have an increased risk of anal carcinoma with similar histological characteristics. This clinical phenomenon is interpreted as a multifocal field effect of cancer-causing agents on epithelium of common embryological origin (Cooper, Patchefsky, and Marks, 1979). As we shall see, cervical carcinoma has been linked to early sexual intercourse and multiple partners. Whatever carcinogens are involved in that process may also act on other epithelial tissues of the same embryonic origin. Hence, chronic anal intercourse may contribute to increased cancer risk in an analogous fashion with multiple-partner vaginal intercourse.

Risk Factors for Gynecological Cancers

Even though risk factors can be identified through epidemiological investigation, these factors cannot necessarily be construed as causal ones (Berg and Lampe, 1981). The term "risk factor" reflects the relatively recent notion that cancer is the end result of the probable interaction of various factors, and it is particularly relevant in the discussion of gynecological cancer. We do not understand the mechanism by which most of these identified factors act in order to increase risk. And the total absence of such risk factors in any particular case does not mean that the individual is not at true risk or that cancer will not develop.

Since the focus of our discussion is on the contribution of behavior to cancer incidence and progression, we will concentrate on evidence linking various sexual life-style factors with neoplasia. Alterations in the body resulting from pregnancy, childbirth, and lactation are clearly different from changes arising from exogenous exposure to chemical carcinogens. However, such somatic changes are considered modifying factors that affect cancer risk. For example, pregnancy and childbirth seem to play a protective role in the development of breast, ovarian, and endometrial cancers, these diseases being less prevalent in women who have had children early in life than in those who have had no children. This relationship with breast cancer is particularly obvious, breast cancer in women who have borne children being progressively less likely to occur as age at first pregnancy drops. A terminated pregnancy does not appear to have a similarly protective effect; therefore, the protective effect produced by full-term delivery may be somehow related to the hormonal trigger to lactate. However, there is little evidence that lactation as such has a protective effect, since nursing an infant is not associated with lower breast cancer risk. Hormones and tumor response are considered in detail in Chapter Six and will not be discussed to any extent here.

The most clear-cut relationship observed between behavior and cancer incidence involves cervical cancer and the character of sexual intercourse (age at onset, number of sexual partners, sexual hygiene, type of contraceptive used, and so on). But other forms of cancer, such as endometrial cancer, also appear to have a behavioral risk component—in this case, chronic use of exogenous estrogen.

Projected statistics from the American Cancer Society (1985) estimate that deaths from cervical cancer in 1985 represent approximately 1.5 percent of all cancer deaths in the United States. However, as Berg and Lampe (1981) point out, it is difficult to generate valid incidence or mortality rates for endometrial or cervical cancer because of the unknown numbers of intact uteri in the population at large or in particular subgroups. That is, we do not know the true population at risk—those who have not had a previous hysterectomy and therefore are at risk for developing these cancers in their lifetime. Therefore, we cannot accurately project risk estimates based on known population statistics. Nevertheless, Doll and Peto (1981) estimate that cancers of the breast, endometrium, and ovary combined represent approximately 13 percent of all cancer deaths in the United States, and possibly half of these could be prevented by ultimately controllable behavioral and environmental risk factors. If we add 1 percent controllable cervical cancer, possibly 7 percent of all these gynecological cancers could be prevented if known or suspected risk factors were altered. Other factors, such as dietary ones, probably contribute to some forms of gynecological cancer. Therefore, the proportion of cancers preventable by dietary modification (discussed in the second section of this chapter) may potentially overlap with preventable cancers as a function of altered sexual behavior.

Cancers of the Vagina, Endometrium, and Ovary. Primary cancer of the vagina is a relatively rare malignancy, comprising 1–2 percent of all gynecological cancer (Dolan, 1978) and found most commonly in older women (average age reported by Dolan as sixty-two). Etiologically, the main predisposing factor in the development of vaginal carcinoma *in situ*, as well as invasive cancer of the site (a more common occurrence), is previous treatment for cancer of the cervix.

The ratio of invasive vaginal cancer to invasive cervical cancer has been reported as approximately 1:3 (Berg and Lampe, 1981). This ratio may be changing, perhaps because the incidence of invasive cervical cancer is dropping while the incidence of invasive vaginal cancer is not. Whereas cervical cancer incidence has been declining, vaginal cancer has increased, so that the proportionate risk for vaginal cancer has increased over time (Berg and Lampe, 1981).

Poor hygiene appears to be associated with risk for cancer of the vagina. And both the age incidence of invasive vaginal cancer and the mortality curve for cervical cancer are quite similar (higher incidence and mortality in the older age groups and among certain population subgroups, such as black women). Both incidence and mortality curves are derived from population data bases containing individuals who receive inadequate gynecological screening.

Postmenopausal bleeding, bloody or purulent vaginal discharge, and pain are common complaints at diagnosis in cases of vaginal cancer of all cell types. The average duration of such symptoms is frequently prolonged—for example, longer than six months; and, again, underscreened and undermonitored populations most frequently present with the signs of late disease (Dolan, 1978).

Endometrial cancers are among the most curable of malignancies if diagnosed before regional spread. Prolonged and abnormal estrogen stimulation is a major risk factor for cancer at this site, risk being greater when dose level has been high. At the same time, carcinomas associated with exogenous estrogen intake tend to be well differentiated; that is, more normal appearing, less aggressive, and hence more curable: "They have an excellent prognosis with a low rate of recurrence; it seems as if most required the exogenous estrogen for growth" (Berg and Lampe, 1981, p. 435).

Following the "iatrogenic epidemic of the 1970s" ("iatrogenic" signifying disease as a result of treatment prescribed), estrogen has been prescribed less frequently; and when it is prescribed, the doses are lower. These changes have reduced endometrial cancer risk to pre-1970s level (Jick, Walter, and Rothman, 1980). Before this risk contributed by medical prescription was fully recognized, endogenous production of estrogen was focused on as the major causative factor. Hyperfunctioning ovaries, including hormone-producing ovarian tumors, were clearly associated with endometrial carcinoma.

Obesity is an additional risk factor, with adipose tissue associated with higher levels of estrogen. An estrogen precursor is transformed to biologically active estrogen by the biochemical process termed aromatization, and this transformation occurs in large measure within fatty tissues of the body. In addition, because of the obvious association with unopposed estrogen, nulliparity (lack of offspring), late menopause, and menstrual irregularity also constitute risk factors for endometrial cancer. Higher social class has also been associated with cancer of this site, presumably because of increased use of prescribed estrogens among women in this social stratum (Austin and Roe, 1979). Finally, Berg and Lampe (1981) point out that there is undoubtedly an interaction effect of exogenous and endogenous estrogens. Mack, Pike, and Henderson (1976) found that chronic use of exogenous estrogens increased the risk of endometrial cancer among obese women by more than fourfold.

As with vaginal cancer, the most common physical complaint for women subsequently diagnosed with endometrial cancer is postmenopausal or other abnormal bleeding, although occasionally abdominal or lower back pain is an associated complaint (Salazar, 1978). As mentioned earlier, especially if a major causative factor is the use of prescribed estrogen, endometrial cancer is highly curable by surgery, frequently in combination with radiotherapy treatment.

In contrast, the prognosis for ovarian cancer is rather

poor. Because of its silent growth pattern and inaccessible character, most patients present with advanced disease. Although ovarian cancer is third in frequency of gynecological tumors, it is the most fatal among the most common of these cancers. Incidence has risen in the last twenty years to approximately seventeen cases per 100,000 population, and 60 percent of ovarian tumors occur in women between forty and sixty years old.

Although the cause or causes of ovarian cancer have not been definitely established, some predisposing factors have been determined. Ovarian carcinomas are more likely to occur in women who have no children or few children, or whose children were born when the mothers were in their thirties or forties (Rubin and Bennett, 1978). Whether low parity is a result of ovarian abnormality preceding frank cancer development, or whether malignancy develops as a result of "incessant ovulation" in the absence of pregnancy or oral contraceptives is still under discussion (Berg and Lampe, 1981). "Of course, the bottom line for either explanation is that the fewer children a woman has had and the older she is, the greater is her risk for ovarian cancer" (Berg and Lampe, 1981, p. 438). A family history of gynecological cancer is also frequently present in patients under treatment for ovarian tumor.

Typical presentation leading to diagnosis of ovarian cancer is pelvic or abdominal mass, accompanied by swelling, pressure, and abdominal discomfort. Again, the onset of ovarian cancer is insidious, and symptoms of pain and other symptoms referable to metastatis and advanced disease often appear within a few months' time.

Other than childbearing pattern, there are few behavioral implications to be drawn related to cancer at this site. There is little that one can do about family history, age, or, in many cases, infertility. And again, whether infertility and low parity are contributive to or a result of subclinical abnormality is very unclear at this point.

Cancer of the Cervix. Incidence of invasive cervical cancer ranks sixth for malignancy in women, although it is only the ninth most common form of cancer death (Berg and Lampe, 1981). However, the incidence is much higher in low socioeconomic groups (blacks and Hispanics), and much lower in nuns, Jewish women, and women who live in nonurban areas. As early as 1842, a clear difference in susceptibility to cervical cancer was noted among cloistered religious women as compared with married females (Hulka, 1982). Other groups who practice strict, monogamous sexual behavior and experience low incidence of veneral disease (for example, Mormons, Jews, and Amish women) also have much lower cervical cancer rates than the population at large.

In contrast, high-risk groups include women who are prostitutes or otherwise have multiple sex partners and experience sexual intercourse beginning early in life—specifically, before the age of seventeen (Hulka, 1982). Age at first pregnancy has been substituted in a number of studies for age at first intercourse (the latter presumably not reliably reported), and the same association has been found. Women reporting earlier pregnancies tend to have higher rates of cervical cancer. Baron and Richart (1971) suggest that pregnancy may have a promotional effect on cervical malignancy previously initiated by early sexual activity.

As mentioned earlier, cervical cancer rates are higher among blacks and Hispanics (almost double the rates for blacks compared to whites), but when socioeconomic status is controlled, the difference between blacks and whites drops out. As Hulka (1982) points out, this social-class distinction may be a proxy for more specific risks generated by particular activities or sexual life-style in these groups—activities such as male promiscuity, or what is referred to in the literature as the "male factor." Consequently, at least in some societies, a woman's cervical cancer risk may be more dependent on her partner's than on her own sexual behavior: "Male sexual behavior, particularly in relation to prostitution, may account for two hitherto unexplained features of the epidemiology of this disease—the extremely high incidence in Latin America and the decline in mortality this century" (Skegg, Corwin, Paul, and Doll, 1982, p. 581). According to Skegg and associates, the high incidence of cervical cancer in Latin America may be a function of *machismo* and the protected status of females in Latin America, forcing males to resort to the use of prostitutes, who may be harboring the infectious agent. The decline in mortality, found especially in the United States and England, may be tied to a more liberalized sexual attitude in both males and females, so that younger males may have less involvement with prostitutes than older generations had.

The importance of the "male factor" is also suggested by the high mortality in wives of males who have occupations that require long absences from home (Beral, 1974). Buckley, Harris, Doll, and Williams (1981) have reported the results of an interview study with husbands of women who were diagnosed with cervical cancer and who reported having sex only with their husbands. A matched control sample of males also were interviewed. The husbands of the cervical cancer patients reported significantly more sexual partners and an earlier age at first intercourse than the husbands in the control group. Although Buckley and associates acknowledge the possibility of bias in their study (for example, the women could have underreported their own sexual experience), they believe that their findings support the notion of a sexually transmitted, infectious, etiological agent; and the "male factor" as source of infection is a viable possibility.

When one considers this high-risk population as a whole—poor, promiscuous, lack of hygiene, early sexual activity, early first pregnancy—the total picture is one of stressful lifestyle, accompanied by poverty and presumably high levels of life stresses. There is strong evidence that in fact cervical cancer is a viral disease, and herpes simplex virus II has been implicated repeatedly as possibly playing a contributive or causative role. And there is a large literature (see, for example, Jemmott and Locke, 1984) linking susceptibility to infectious disease with social/environmental stress and poor coping ability on the part of the individual.

The herpes virus is capable of infecting both male and female genital tracts. Herpes simplex virus II is biologically different from herpes simplex virus I, the virus that causes the common "cold sore." Transmission of herpes simplex virus II during sexual activity has been demonstrated in laboratory animals

(Nahmias, Naib, and Highsmith, 1967) and has been clinically confirmed by Rawls and associates (1971), who have reported transmission of this virus from sixteen males to 78 percent of their susceptible female partners. A number of studies have shown that cervical cancer cells possess herpes simplex virus II antigens, and infectious herpes simplex virus II has been isolated from cervical cancer cells grown in culture (Aurelian, Strandberg, and Marcus, 1974). Furthermore, longitudinal studies following women with herpes simplex virus II have demonstrated a statistically higher incidence of cervical cancer in the cases followed (Nahmias, Naib, and Josey, 1973). These and other studies (Graham, Rawls, Swanson, and McCurtis, 1982; Catalano and Johnson, 1971) have produced strong evidence for the role of viral transmission in the induction of cervical carcinoma.

The viral and immunological evidence suggests that increased risk for cervical cancer may be mediated by central nervous system immune pathways modulated by life stress and disordered social systems. Animal studies and clinically based research strongly indicate that the absence of intact social networks, as well as other forms of social stress, has a deleterious effect on the organism's ability to withstand further insult, including the invasion of viral organisms. The host—animal or human—then becomes vulnerable to infection as a result of hormone alteration and immune suppression.

Chapters Five, Six, and Seven of this book discuss in depth this more direct effect of behavior on host status. It is sufficient here to suggest that there may be a highly plausible biological pathway explaining increased risk of cervical cancer—perhaps virally induced—in the population subgroups already identified as at high risk for this disease

Behavioral Implications. Socially, it is less than feasible to proscribe poverty, poor hygiene, ignorance, estrogen use, and adolescent sexual activity—although at the level of medical-social policy and educational planning, this level of risk can certainly be addressed. On an individual level, however,there is evidence that certain barrier forms of contraception may play a protective role in cervical cancer. For example, Wright and colleagues (1978) found that in a large sample of women the incidence rate of cervical cancer in diaphragm users was much lower than the rates in oral contraceptive users or in those who used intrauterine devices. They also found that diaphragm users were less likely to have had intercourse at an early age and had fewer sexual partners than the comparison groups. "After adjusting for the effects of these variables, however, the risk of cervical neoplasia in diaphragm users was still only about one fourth that in the users of the other methods" (Wright and others, 1978, p. 273).

Richardson and Lyon (1981) found a substantial degree of disease regression in cervical cancer patients whose only "treatment" was the instruction that their partners use the condom (another barrier device) during sexual intercourse. Hulka (1982), in her review of risk factors in cervical cancer, reports that a number of studies have shown a lower incidence of cervical cancer among diaphragm users and a higher incidence among those who chose to take steroid hormones in the form of birth control pills. She cautions, however, that a selection bias could be operative here. That is, certain types of women—conservative, methodical, future oriented, organized—may select a diaphragm; therefore, this selection may simply be a surrogate measure of a total life-style including "conservative" sexual activity but extending beyond that area to their lives as a whole. Nevertheless, the evidence for viral infection cannot be ignored, and some form of barrier contraceptive could play a protective role in this regard.

Screening in High-Risk Populations. Although we will be discussing the issue of cancer screening in general in Chapter Four, the decline in cervical cancer mortality can be in large part directly attributable to more universal screening by Pap smear and therefore to the diagnosis of cervical cancer at an earlier stage. But, as we shall see in Chapter Four, there are pockets of underscreened populations—elderly women and the minority disadvantaged—where cervical cancer is still diagnosed when the disease is unnecessarily advanced. Unlike other forms of cancer—including other types of gynecological cancer, such as ovarian carcinoma—cervical cancer might prove to be curable in virtually all cases if screening were universal. Although there is still controversy over the necessary frequency of Pap testing over a lifetime, all would agree that an initial two negative tests for every female—particularly those who are sexually active—is mandatory. In fact, since sexual activity apparently constitutes the necessary "risk behavior," it has been suggested that even sexually active adolescents should be routinely screened. Hein, Schreiber, Cohen, and Koss (1977) found a high percentage of atypical cervical cells, as well as early precancerous changes, in a sample of sexually active girls, twelve to sixteen years old. Since all patients screened were asymptomatic but sexually active, no clinically obvious symptoms distinguished the negative from the positive cytology cases. "The data suggest that cervical cytologic screening should be incorporated into the routine examination of sexually active female adolescents" (Hein, Schreiber, Cohen, and Koss, 1977, p. 123).

The fact that these girls were screened in a youth detention center again underscores the association of premature and possibly promiscuous sexual behavior with other aspects of social disorder and disorganization in these individuals' lives. But there are points of intervention that may be behaviorally feasible, and screening—on admission to institutions such as hospitals, clinics, or detention centers—represents a preventive intervention that can potentially save lives.

Acquired Immune Deficiency, Malignancy, and Sexual Life-Style

Acquired immune deficiency syndrome (AIDS) has received a great deal of attention in recent years, attention that is apparently justified. As a society we seem to be witnessing the development of a new, lethal syndrome whose viral cause is now known and whose mortality rate is essentially 100 percent. And cases of reported AIDS are doubling every thirteen months. This syndrome is relevant for us to consider here because this apparently irreversible acquired defect in cell-mediated immunity predisposes the individual to severe infections and/or unusual malignancies, such as Kaposi's sarcoma (KS). Historically, this cancer was first characterized in 1872 by Moriz Kaposi, who described three fatal cases seen in elderly Viennese men. In patients with classical KS, dark-blue or purple-brown plaques or nodules occur, most commonly on the extremities. The incidence of KS is highest in elderly Jewish and Italian males but is also quite evident in some equatorial African countries. The KS that appears in Africans affects younger as well as older patients; the juvenile form is more aggressive than cases seen in European counterparts. The KS that appears in AIDS victims is also of an aggressive variety and appears among younger patients.

At first AIDS was believed confined to populations of male homosexuals; but other populations, such as intravenous drug users and persons born in Haiti, later became identified as at risk. Very soon in the disease identification process, the concept of a transmissible agent became paramount. With the localization of AIDS as present among hemophiliacs, the assumption of disease transmissibility became accepted as most probable. One of the most publicized of transmission-related cases concerned a twenty-month-old child from San Francisco who developed an immune deficiency syndrome identical to cases of AIDS in adults. The infant had received multiple blood transfusions while hospitalized for an unrelated disorder. After the AIDS-like syndrome developed in the child, it was determined that one of the nineteen previously healthy donors had subsequently developed AIDS and died of the disease (Editorial, *Journal of the American Medical Association*, 1983).

Such incidents provide strong support for the notion of transmissible infectious agents in the AIDS process. Epidemiological observations suggest that AIDS is caused by an infectious agent transmitted sexually or by exposure to contaminated blood or blood products. Among the agents studied as causes of AIDS are the retroviruses. Such viruses contain an enzyme that copies RNA into DNA and thus has RNA as its genetic material. Gallo and colleagues at the National Cancer Institute (Popovic, Sarngadharan, Read, and Gallo, 1984; Gallo and others, 1984; Schupbach and others, 1984; Marx, 1985) have isolated a retrovirus, human T-cell lymphotropic virus, designated HTLV-III, as a likely infectious agent for AIDS development. Antibodies to HTLV-III virus have been reported in 90 to 100 percent of AIDS patients—indicating that they probably have been infected with this virus. The HTLV-III targets and destroys the immune system's T-helper cells, lymphocytes that help other immune cells carry out their function. The immune depression of AIDS patients is mainly caused by severe loss of T-helper cells.

The study of viruses linked with AIDs continues to advance rapidly. Other research teams in addition to Gallo's NCI group have now characterized the nucleotide sequences of gene material linked to the disease. Researchers at the Pasteur Institute in Paris (Barré-Sinoussi and others, 1983) have described what they term "lymphadenopathy-associated virus" derived from the lymph nodes of a French homosexual male with chronic lymphadenopathy. And Levy and his colleagues (1984) have reported the sequence of a virus they call "AIDS-associated retrovirus" (ARV). There is general agreement among all these researchers that, despite different names, these are all variants of the same virus.

Life-Style as Risk Factor. As indicated earlier, this current epidemic of AIDS has not been limited to homosexual males. Over 17 percent of the cases reported by Haverkos and Curran (1982) were heterosexual men or women (or men whose sexual orientation was unknown). Fifty-six percent of these were intravenous drug abusers, and outbreaks of AIDS with Kaposi's sarcoma have occurred in other population subgroups—Haitians and hemophiliacs.

Sonnabend, Witkin, and Purtilo (1983) have likened the final stage of AIDS to a wasting disorder resembling chronic graft-versus-host disease. Related to increased risk among homosexuals, antigenic lymphocytes in the semen passing into an already immune-compromised host could alter the regulation of the immune apparatus, precipitating a graft-versus-host disease. In the final disease phase, the host cannot immunologically control the cells infected with virus. This alteration of immune response may be controlled by T-suppressor lymphocytes, by immune complexes blocking immune control, by autoantibodies developed in response to sperm "invasion," and by selective killing of T-helper cells by HTLV-III or related viruses. Sonnabend and colleagues suggest that these immune defects may correlate with sexual promiscuity, but the mechanism of transmission of this immunosuppressive disease is still not fully understood. Transmission occurs by way of virally infected lymphocytes, with the causal virus clearly having been identified in both blood and semen. However, while the virus is also recoverable from saliva, there is currently no good evidence of spread by this route.

Findings from a study reported by Stahl and associates (1982) suggest that healthy homosexuals may be at more risk than heterosexual males for developing opportunistic infections and other diseases associated with immune suppression. They examined immunological functioning in homosexual men with Kaposi's sarcoma, homosexual men with hyperplastic lymphadenopathy, healthy homosexual males, and a group of heterosexual males with Kaposi's sarcoma. Significant immunological abnormalities were observed in all three homosexual groups— including the "healthy" subgroup. The most severely compromised were the homosexuals with Kaposi's sarcoma. The next most compromised were the homosexuals with lymphadenopathy, and the least compromised (but still abnormal) were the immunological responses in homosexuals who were healthy. The heterosexual subgroup—depite having been diagnosed with Kaposi's sarcoma—showed essentially normal immune function. Of particular note among the homosexual groups was the striking inversion of normal T-helper to T-suppressor subpopulations. In general, T-suppressor cells outnumbered T-helper cells (the reverse of what is typically found in normal subjects) and presumably played an important role in suppressing immune control over infectious agents.

Stahl and associates suggest that infections and drug use should be considered as causes of immune abnormality in these homosexual subgroups. Homosexual men frequently develop immunosuppressive, sexually transmitted diseases such as cytomegalovirus (CMV). Alternatively, the common use of inhalant drugs, such as amyl nitrite and butyl nitrite, and other psychotomimetic drugs (Khansari, Whitten, and Fudenberg, 1984) may play a contributive role. However, few data currently exist regarding the effect of these drugs on immunological status, and both epidemiological and laboratory studies are under way to examine the association between their use and immunological status.

Behavioral Implications. Findings suggesting the particular at-risk status of homosexuals—even those still healthy—prompted Sonnabend, Witkin, and Purtilo (1983) to hazard behavioral intervention recommendations in order to reduce this risk. These recommendations are clearly preliminary, since we do not know the entire causal sequence of events surrounding AIDS and its various manifestiations, including Kaposi's sarcoma.

Acquired immune deficiency undoubtedly has multiple co-factors—among them, malnutrition, the use of various recreational and medical drugs, as well as causal viral infections. Some of these factors could be playing a contributive role in the outbreak of AIDS in Haitian and hemophiliac subpopulations. And some of these causal factors are more controllable than others. But to the extent that sexual practice plays a major role, behavioral implications can be drawn. As Sonnabend and co-workers urge, two rational steps in preventing the development of AIDS and its associated disorders would be to restrict sexual activity to the smallest number of partners possible and to use condoms during sexual contact.

Sonnabend and colleagues also suggest that higher-risk, highly promiscuous homosexual males should receive immunological screening to examine markers of immune impairment, such as an inverted T-suppressor/T-helper cell ratio. Such screening could facilitate early recognition of the immune deficiency syndrome and would allow intervention during this precursor acquisition phase.

Diet and Cancer Risk

The following case illustrates a possible association between chronic nutritional deficiency and esophageal cancer in a low socioeconomic population.

James N., a sixty-seven-year-old impoverished male, was brought into an inner-city hospital emergency ward by a social worker who infrequently provided social services to males reporting to one of the city's four residential shelters for the destitute. James reportedly had not eaten for several days, although food was available at the shelter, and had lost over twenty pounds in the previous two months. On physical examination he was found to have a persistent cough, with left vocal cord paralysis from recurrent nerve palsy. Barium swallow, laryngoscopy, and bronchoscopy revealed malignant lesions to the upper esophagus, with histopathological findings of moderately undifferentiated epidermal carcinoma present. On further examination metastatic spread to the mediastinum lymph nodes, lung, and pleura was discovered, with probably additional spread to the liver. Since prognosis was so poor, only palliative treatment was instituted. The patient received radiation treatment, but esophageal perforation occurred as a result of the extent of lesions. The patient rapidly deteriorated, and death ensued two months after initial diagnosis.

Poverty, Nutritional Deficit, and Cancer Risk

A number of recent reports (Berg, Ross, and Latourette, 1977; Mettlin, 1980; Pottern and others, 1981; Ziegler and others, 1981) provide evidence for an association between poverty, poor dietary habits, and cancer risk. For example, Pottern and Ziegler and their colleagues conducted a case-control study in the Washington, D.C., area to determine why excessively high mortality rates from esophageal cancer were occurring among the black population in that city. The age-adjusted annual death rate in Washington, D.C., for nonwhite males, 1970–1975, was 28.6/100,000, far in excess of the national rate of 12.4/100,000. In the survey the relatives of 120 esophageal cancer patients who died during 1975 to 1977, and next of kin of 250 black males who died from other diseases, were interviewed. These investigators found that the least nourished third of the study population (for example, low ingestion of meat or fish, dairy products, fruits, and vegetables, coupled with least number of meals per day and lowest relative weight) had twice the risk of esophageal cancer mortality than the most nourished third. This association of poor nutrition and cancer risk continued to hold even after alcohol consumption and tobacco use were controlled for. However, alcohol consumption increased the risk for cancer over and above poor nutrition: "Since poor nutrition is a risk factor for esophageal cancer, it is conceivable that alcohol increases risk, in part, by reducing nutrient intake. Beer, wine, and hard liquor provide a source of daily caloric needs and consequently reduce appetite, but provide almost none of the daily requirements for micronutrients and protein" (Ziegler and others, 1981, p. 1205).

The role of excessive alcohol consumption found in this study may not be generalizable to the nonwhite population as a whole. Data from another survey, a health and nutrition survey carried out between 1971 and 1974 by the National Center for Health Statistics, do not indicate that blacks are heavier drinkers than whites (Mettlin, 1980). In fact, a number of additional surveys (Johnson, Armor, Polich, and Stambul, 1977; Russell and Welte, 1979) reflect just the opposite—that is, that blacks are more likely to abstain from alcohol use than whites are.

However, as we saw in Chapter One, blacks are at greater risk for cancers at various sites—and tend to die sooner than their white counterparts with the same diagnosis. Poverty and nutritional deficit in the disadvantaged—black or white—appear to be major risk factors across studies. Berg, Ross, and Latourette (1977) compared the survival rates of sixty or more indigent cancer patients, seen during 1940 to 1969, with those of nonindigent cancer patients in the same hospital. For all cancers the indigent patients had a lower survival rate than nonindigent patients. Quality of care was not an issue here, since indigent and "clinic pay" patients received essentially identical treatment. Survival rates of another group of patients in the same hospital—private patients, who received different treatment—were not materially different from the survival rates of clinic pay patients. The main problems associated with poor outcome were high mortality from other causes and "excess cancer mortality not accounted for by stage differences, particularly among patients who should have had five-year survival rates between 40 percent and 70 percent" (p. 467). In this latter group, cancer recurred earlier and more often among the nonpaying, indigent patients.

Berg, Ross, and Latourette speculate that host differences associated with poverty accounted for many of the black-white and income-level differences that occurred. In addition, they speculate that blacks may have lower survival rates than whites because they are immunologically less resistant to the spread of cancer or have more aggressive histological forms of neoplasia, or because of host differences that determine differential biological response to treatment. Possibly, these investigators suggest, alterations in host characteristics among the disadvantaged (black or white) can be linked to alcoholism or nutritional deficit: "There is a tendency for cancer cells to implant themselves where tissue is abnormal, and perhaps the connective tissue of the malnourished, like a bowel anastomosis, is a favorable site for cancer growth" (p. 476). Conceivably, host differences such as these could be reversible, increasing the chances for survival among the socially disadvantaged.

Specific Dietary Components in Cancer Prevention and Risk

Americans are sometimes accused of being a cancerphobic people, and probably this tendency is nowhere more apparent than our preoccupation with possible cancer-causing agents in the diet. Frequent news reports of saccharin scares and the like are evidence of this preoccupation and serve to reinforce the public's concern about the possible lethal consequences of what it ingests. Indeed, a recent issue of *Science* (Ames, 1983) contains an article that carefully describes the evidence linking our natural foodstuff (from black pepper and mushrooms to corn and peanut butter) with a large variety of mutagens and carcinogens that are naturally derived. The reader finishes the article with the impression that "everything" causes cancer and undoubtedly wonders how he or she has escaped the disease so far.

In that article Ames describes probable mechanisms underlying mutagenic and carcinogenic processes, one of which is the cellular release of free oxygen radicals contributing to DNA damage. These endogenous oxygen radicals arise in large part as a product of cellular metabolism, and their damaging effects are countered by many types of enzymes that protect cells from "oxidative damage" (p. 1259). As Ames points out, there are additionally a number of small molecules in our diet that function as antioxidating agents—among them vitamin E, beta carotene, and ascorbic acid.

Ames concludes by stressing that no human diet can be entirely free of mutagens and carcinogens and that, beyond identifying their presence in the diet, one needs to consider risks and benefits of removing such factors. For example, food preservatives carry some cancer risk. However, the possible harm of ingesting food that is contaminated with the bacteria and other toxins that are prevented by sodium nitrite and other additives must be considered. "Depite all of these risks, it should be emphasized that the overall trend in life expectancy in the United States is continuing steadily upward" (p. 1261).

In the following discussion of diet and cancer, we will primarily consider human epidemiological evidence related to diet and cancer risk—since generalizations drawn from animal research on dietary effects and applied to the human condition are always problematic, in part because of longevity differences between species and the probable multiple causes of cancer in man. Furthermore, although many dietary components, including micronutrients such as Vitamin A and selenium, are hypothesized to play a role in cancer prevention, the strongest human evidence for the risk effects of diet concerns the macronutrients fat and fiber. Therefore, we will concentrate on these two substances. Of course, the behavioral implications related particularly to fat consumption versus the implications related to possible preventive effects of various vitamins and minerals are in themselves problematic. It is presumed, at least, that individuals are more willing to add things to their diet than to remove habitual dietary components. It is one matter to ingest vitamin capsules; it is quite another matter to reduce one's dietary consumption of fat by half. As we shall see, the latter requires a rather massive alteration in food shopping and preparing, as well as shifting palatability requirements. All this change calls for long-term commitment and great motivation to carry out.

Dietary Fat, Obesity, and Cancer Risk. The importance of general nutrition related to tumor susceptibility was revealed over forty years ago by Tannenbaum's (1942) experiments on mice, which showed that restricting the intake of food without modifying the proportion of the individual components could reduce the incidence of spontaneous breast, lung, and other cancers by half. The underfed mice grew to half the size of the normally fed control group but were sleek and active, appeared in perfect health, and lived on the average longer than the controls.

The association between excess weight and cancer mortality has been confirmed by the American Cancer Society (Lew and Garfinkel, 1979). However, the association between obesity and general cancer mortality was not very striking in that survey. It was most consistent for women—more specifically, for endometrial and gall bladder cancer in women. This association with endometrial cancer is relatively easy to understand, since, as we saw earlier, endometrial cancer can be produced by excessive exposure to estrogen. And the only natural estrogens to which women are exposed after menopause are made from adrenal hormones in adipose tissue. In fact, after menopause the level of estrogen in the blood is directly proportional to the degree of adiposity. "Apart from cancer of the endometrium, no other type of cancer has been related so definitely to overnutrition or to a specific component of the common American or European diet, except insofar as the high standard of nutrition in childhood also advances the age at menarche, which, in view of the association that exists between early menarche and breast cancer risk, will presumably increase the subsequent risk of breast cancer" (Doll and Peto, 1981, p. 1234).

Even though Doll and Peto speak of "overnutrition" as a cancer risk factor, a report by the Committee on Diet, Nutrition, and Cancer (1982) of the National Academy of Sciences, indicates that neither the experiments with animals nor the epidemiological studies allow clear interpretation of the effects of total caloric intake on risk of cancer. The experimental studies failed to distinguish between the effects of total caloric reduction and the effects of the reduction of the specific subset, such as dietary fat. "The studies conducted in animals show that a reduction in total food intake decreases the age-specific incidence of cancer. The evidence is less clear for human beings'' (p. 1-4). However, the committee concluded that, of all the dietary components it considered, the evidence is most supportive for a causal relationship between fat intake and the occurrence of cancer. Dietary fat appears to have a promoting effect on tumor development. For example, the development of colon cancer may be enhanced by the increased secretion of bile acids and steroids that are associated with high levels of fat intake. However, since the underlying mechanisms involved in such a promotion process are not well understood, a role for dietary fat in cancer initiation cannot be ruled out at this time.

In animal studies an increase in fat intake from 10 percent to 40 percent of total calories consumed increases the tumor incidence in various tissues, and evidence from epidemiological studies shows that cancers of the breast and colon in particular increase with increasing consumption of dietary fats. Data from animal studies also suggest that, when fat intake is relatively low, polyunsaturated fats are more effective in enhancing tumor growth than saturated fats are. However, human data do not allow such a distinction between types of dietary fats. In general, the evidence from both epidemiological and laboratory studies is consistent and demonstrates that dietary fat is a highly probable cancer risk factor.

Dietary Fiber and Cancer Protection. Most studies of dietary fiber have attempted to determine whether high-fiber diets (for example, diets high in whole grain cereal, fruits, and certain fiber-containing vegetables) protect against colorectal cancer. "Fiber," of course, refers to remnants of the cell wall not hydrolyzed by alimentary enzymes. It is found particularly in whole wheat, which contains lignins that pass through the bowel undigested; cellulose, which is partially digested in the large bowel; and various polymers, which are largely degraded and increase the population of certain intestinal bacteria. Findings from case-control and correlational studies have been mixed, some studies suggesting that high-fiber diets afford a protection against colorectal cancer and some suggesting no association. Laboratory studies in which specific fiber components have been isolated show that the consumption of certain fiber ingredients (for example, bran and cellulose) inhibits the experimental induction of colon cancer. Such findings are difficult to compare with epidemiological findings, because epidemiologists generally have been concerned with the effects of ingesting fiber-containing foods rather than specific fiber components. One correlational study with humans (Bingham, Williams, Cole, and James, 1979) suggests that the incidence of colon cancer is inversely related to the intake of one fiber component—the pentosan fraction—found in whole wheat products and other foods. The Committee on Diet, Nutrition, and Cancer (1982) of the National Academy of Sciences concluded that as yet there is no conclusive evidence that fiber in general provides protection against colon or rectal cancer in humans; specific components of fiber may produce a protective effect, but these components have yet to be completely characterized.

Doll and Peto (1981), speculating the mechanism by which fiber might effect cancer reduction, suggest that such a component or components might do so "by decreasing the length of time stools remain in the bowel, by decreasing the concentration of carcinogens in stools (through increasing their bulk), or perhaps by altering the total numbers or proportions of different bacterial species in the bowel, some of which may produce or destroy carcinogenic metabolites" (p. 1230).

Bingham and associates (1979), using food tables specifying amounts of various components of fiber in certain foods, correlated dietary fiber consumption with colon cancer mortality by geographical region. The findings revealed an inverse relationship only between the pentose fiber content in the diet and mortality from colon cancer. Pentose polymers are particularly plentiful in unrefined cereal fiber and to a lesser extent in various vegetables (but not in potatoes). As in any geographical study, however, other unknown factors could be playing a controlling or contributing role, and the exact relationship between particular fibers and cancer risk will not be known until intervention trials are completed.

Dietary Trials in Cancer Prevention. Based on the above epidemiological and laboratory evidence, human trials manipulating dietary fat and fiber are currently under way. The weight of the evidence suggests that dietary fat reduction and increased fiber intake—particularly in the form of whole wheat, bran, and other unrefined cereals—should have a cancer-preventive effect. But until randomized clinical trials are performed, this evidence is only suggestive.

Boyd (1985) describes an ongoing Canadian study in which the fat intake of women with breast dysplasia has been reduced to about half that of the usual American diet (typically, 40 percent of total caloric intake as fat), in the hopes of reversing the dysplasia and reducing risk of progression to neoplasia in these women. In order to reduce fat consumption to 20 percent instead of 40 percent of total caloric intake, rather large shifts in buying, cooking, and eating patterns need to be carried out. In the *Alternative Diet Book* (Connor, Connor, Fry, and Warner, 1980), which aims at such extensive fat reduction, the authors suggest a gradual dietary shift, carried out in three separate phases. Phase 1 consists of deleting egg yolk, butterfat, lard, organ meat, skin of poultry and fish, and visible fat from meat; decreasing table salt; and substituting margarine for butter, skim milk for whole, and egg whites for whole eggs. Phase 2 includes reduction of meat consumption to no more than six ounces a day; meatless lunches; and further reductions of fat, cheese, and salt. Phase 3 has been mastered when the diet contains mainly cereals, fruits, and vegetables; meat is eaten sparingly, as a condiment; and only low-cholesterol cheeses are consumed. A sample daily menu includes orange juice, cereal, and rye toast for breakfast; lentil soup, fresh fruit, and bran muffins for lunch; and sukiyaki with rice, sliced peach salad, and sliced cheesecake (made with egg whites and low-fat yogurt) for dinner.

It is understandable that such a diet, when undertaken not for just a short period of time but for many years, is exceedingly difficult to manage. Yet Boyd (1985) has reported acceptable compliance rates in the above-mentioned trial, measured by both reported fat intake and serum cholesterol values. However, he also points out that this ongoing trial is quite labor intensive and that the subjects, a relatively small number of women, are being monitored closely and given extensive help in meal preparation and general diet maintenance. The major side effect in Boyd's study has been the inability of some of the women to replace the energy that they would have gained from fat with energy derived from carbohydrate sources. Therefore, the maintenance of body weight has been a problem for some subjects. Nevertheless, even though this trial has not yet demonstrated any biological effects of the fat reduction related to cancer risk, it does demonstrate the feasibility of carrying out such trials in human populations.

The control group in Boyd's trial is composed of women with breast dysplasia and counseled to adhere to the recommended diet for Canadians found in *Canada's Food Guide*, which until recently did not emphasize fat reduction. As Bright-See and Levy (1985) point out, however, this approach to a placebo or control arm of the dietary trial may not be feasible in the future, since the latest version of the *Food Guide* includes a recommendation to "decrease your total fat intake." In fact, this dietary fat reduction appears to be occurring in both Canada and the United States as the popular press highlights the possible importance of dietary fat reduction.

In addition to this particular fat reduction trial and a larger one initiated in 1984 by the National Cancer Institute in the United States—both aimed at the prevention or control of breast cancer in high-risk women—pilot studies of the role of dietary fiber in the prevention of colon cancer are being conducted (Bright-See and Levy, 1985). A high-fiber snack (HFS), supplying nearly 20 grams of dietary fiber from wheat bran per daily intake, and a low-fiber snack (LFS), with approximately 3.5 grams of fiber per daily intake, have been developed to study the effect of high fiber in the recurrence of colon polyps. Thus far, these products have been tested for acceptability, side effects, and effects on other dietary variables in a pilot group of healthy adults. Compliance—assessed by self-report, as well as urinary riboflavin output—has been acceptable. Several health parameters (such as weight and blood pressure) have been monitored. The investigators found that serum ferritin and serum calcium values tended to decrease over the study period because the snacks affected the absorption of these nutrients. Therefore, for long-term intervention these snack products will need to be enriched with both calcium and iron. This finding of undesirable side effects underscores the need for preliminary testing of experimental interventions in the diet area, even with such a "benign" intervention as dietary fiber.

There has also been preliminary work on a fiber-fat intervention trial in Canada. In Boyd's preliminary work, maintenance of total energy intake was a problem for some women in the fat reduction group, and in the preliminary high-fiber/low-fiber snack trial, subjects tended not to compensate for energy in the snacks by decreasing voluntary energy intake. But in the combined fiber/fat intervention, the average total energy intake was stable over a two-month period. Therefore, these two interventions may in fact be complementary, so that compliance in a combined long-term trial may be better than compliance to either diet intervention alone (Bright-See and Levy, 1985).

Behavioral Implications. Obviously, until the results of the above experimental trials are known, all the evidence remains epidemiological and laboratory, with the inherent limits in both these methods. Epidemiological studies showing geographical distributions of cancer incidence related to diet for large populations of subjects can be confounded with unknown factors contributing to the observed associations. Laboratory animal studies often induce tumors by some means or another, and generalization across animal species and tumor systems is inherently limited and problematic. An editorial in the issue of *Science* containing the article cited earlier on dietary carcinogens concludes in the following manner: "When more definitive information is available, it should be possible for prudent people to choose fruits and vegetables that present minimal hazards. In the meantime, there is persuasive evidence that charred meats and rancid fats should not be part of the diet" (Editorial, *Science*, Sept. 23, 1983). Although we have not here discussed *charred* meats and *rancid* fats, we have discussed meat and fat and the implications for cancer risk. Based on the aggregate of what we already know, it would probably be prudent to reduce dietary fat consumption in the standard American diet by 10–15 percent; and based on suggestive epidemiological evidence, daily consumption of foods high in fiber content would also be a reasonable course to pursue. Such diet modification should not be too difficult to accomplish, given a well-designed and implemented public education program.

Role of Nutrition in Cancer Treatment

In the case of cancer patients, the major concern is usually how to increase total energy and nutrient intake in order to override factors suppressing food consumption. Although it has been hypothesized (Copeland and Dudrick, 1976), on the basis of animal studies of underfeeding, that malnutrition may improve a patient's condition, a more plausible hypothesis is that what affects the tumor and its nutritional needs also affects the body as a whole. Malnutrition affects normal cells at the same time that the added burden of the tumor's presence interferes with available nutrients. For example, cancer cells incorporate nitrogen from body tissues. As nitrogen flows in one direction and is "trapped" by the tumor cells, patients move into a negative nitrogen balance, with nitrogen depletion becoming worse as the tumor progresses.

The eating behavior and consequent nutritional status of cancer patients are related to tumor burden or to treatment side effects, such as nausea during chemotherapy. For example, in one study (Donaldson, 1982) overt malnutrition was found in 17 percent of children with newly diagnosed localized tumors and in 37 percent of patients with metastatic disease. In a second, retrospective study of one thousand patients with a variety of neoplastic disorders, significant weight loss occurred in nearly half of the sample (Costa and Donaldson, 1980). Although not all weight loss in cancer patients is simply the result of lower caloric intake, eating difficulties contribute significantly to physical wasting (Bernstein and Treneer, 1985).

The development of nutritional deficit is also not related simply to extent of tumor burden, anatomical site involved, or cell type. Neither is the degree of physical wasting directly associated with the anatomical involvement of tumor. Attempts have been made to identify metabolic effects of cancer cells, but, except for a few ectopic hormones, no tumor "toxin" has been unequivocally identified (Costa and Donaldson, 1980). Patient weight loss in fact is generally attributable to a "negative energy balance," because of decreased caloric intake and increased energy exenditure by the host. "Alterations in protein metabolism include preferential intake of amino acids by the tumor, decreased synthesis of some host tissue proteins, such as muscle tissue, and increased synthesis of other host proteins. Lipid metabolism is seemingly less affected. These metabolic changes result in muscle wasting in adult cancer patients, and failure to grow in pediatric cancer patients. Host tissues are catabolized to meet the nutritional demands of the tumor, and nutritional death may ensue" (DeWys, 1982, p. 721S). Ultimately, the pathological limiting factor is not the nutritional status but the biology of the tumor invading the host (Levine and others, 1982).

In addition to metabolic effects of neoplasia, caloric intake is frequently compromised by nausea, vomiting, and loss of appetite in patients under treatment. These side effects of toxic therapies are sometimes themselves learned behavioral phenomena associated with the treatment context (Bernstein and Treneer, 1985). (See Burish, Levy, and Meyerwitz, 1985, for a thorough examination of treatment-related issues in the area of diet and cancer.)

As a matter of course, nutritional counseling should be provided to cancer patients undergoing treatment. Minor nutritional problems probably can be corrected if the patient is encouraged to eat small, frequent meals throughout the day and new recipes are provided to enhance palatability and ease of food intake (for example, making foods easier to swallow). Family members also can be encouraged to provide a pleasant dining atmosphere. For more seriously ill patients or for patients with acute disturbance, such as postchemotherapy nausea, more specialized interventions are required. For example, supportive feeding of highly nutritious, easily digestible food with vitamin supplements through a nasogastric tube can be provided for patients who have difficulty in swallowing or who have a tumor-associated obstruction. Systematic muscle relaxation in order to counter treatment-associated nausea and vomiting has also proved to be an effective behavioral intervention (Burish, Levy, and Meyerwitz, 1985). There are other kinds of ancillary behavioral techniques that can be used in the service of patient nutritional support. For example, Costa and Donaldson (1980) have discussed the use of techniques such as behavioral shaping and cognitive preparation in support of dietary, mechanical intervention, such as tube feeding.

Summary of Findings and Recommendations

We have tried to draw out preventive implications in our discussion of cancer risk associated with sexuality in all forms—heterosexual as well as homosexual. For the female gynecological cancers, we know most about the prevention, early detection, treatment, and cure of cervical cancer. Thus, the recommendations regarding periodic screening and protection against viral infection and the importance of personal hygiene are fairly straightforward. Our discussion of homosexual practices and sexual promiscuity, associated with AIDS and Kaposi's sarcoma, is much more tentative. The lines of evidence are more circumstantial, although laboratory evidence of immunological disregulation and the antigeneity of sperm bears directly on disease risk in these populations. Perhaps the preventive implications drawn by Sonnabend and colleagues (1983)—namely, that the number of sexual partners be restricted, that condoms be used, and that high-risk males receive immunological screening—should be viewed at this point as interim recommendations until all the facts are in. Given the strong evidence for viral contribution in sexually associated cancers, moderation is probably sound interim advice.

As for diet: We began this chapter with a discussion of the fundamental significance of food consumption, as well as sexual behavior, for the human condition. Although one would probably not want to go so far as to suggest that "you are what you eat," nevertheless, in some basic sense, that is true. Cellular metabolism requires food intake and nourishment; food intake of a certain kind—for example, fat consumption—may promote malignant cell growth. But on a social and cultural level, the taking in of food is rich with symbolic meaning and ritual. As examples of such symbolism, for large numbers of Christians, the sacrifice of the Mass is a communal meal, as well as the reliving of the Last Supper and the taking in of the Body of Christ. For Jews the Passover feast is one of the highest holy days of the religious year, with special food blessed and consumed in a ritualized manner.

The evidence linking diet and cancer is available and suggestive—and some of it worthy of further examination in controlled human trials. Behavioral implications at this point—particularly in the prevention area—are few. Obviously, malnutrition in the disadvantaged, as well as in patient populations, contributes to host risk. But beyond that—with the possible exception of dietary fiber increase and fat reduction—little can be prescribed. The aggregate of the hard evidence does not justify the extent of the public concern related to diet and cancer risk. Only an understanding of the significance of eating behavior within the human social matrix can make understandable the extraordinary public outcry over the possible cancer-causing aspects of our American diet.

4

☒☒☒☒☒☒☒☒☒☒☒☒☒☒☒☒

Progression of Cancer: Role of Screening, Early Detection, and Compliance with Treatment

This chapter is concerned primarily with *indirect* behavioral and social contributors to cancer growth, once the disease is established. For example, if an individual ignores a persistent hoarseness in his voice quality or a gross thickening of a mole on the surface of his skin, and if laryngeal cancer or malignant melanoma is finally diagnosed, it probably will be diagnosed at an advanced stage of disease, where successful treatment and cure are less likely. Although the delay in diagnosis will not directly affect the course and progression of the cancerous growth, it very well may affect the eventual outcome of the disease. Hence, such a behavioral contribution in this case would be considered indirect.

We are concerned here, then, with the early detection of cancer through mass screening, early case finding in the physician's office, and early diagnosis and treatment of pathology. In addition, in a later section of this chapter, we will consider behavioral factors that indirectly affect cancer treatment in general. A major focus will be on patient (or family) compliance with established cancer treatments. But we will also consider related issues: "active noncompliance" or the resorting to unorthodox treatments; "noncompliance" by physicians; the process of informed consent to experimental treatment regimen; and, finally, issues related to the management of the terminally ill.

Reasons for Delays in Seeking Diagnosis

The following passage—from *The Death of Ivan Ilych* (Tolstoy, [1886] 1960, pp. 116, 123)—captures an intrinsic human tendency to normalize experience into the familiar or the known. Schutz (1973) speaks of the process of "typification" in this regard. One perceives a symptom, for example, and explains it or views it as a typical instance of what is already understood.

> It's a good thing I'm a bit of an athlete. Another man might have been killed, but I merely knocked myself, just here; it hurts when it's touched, but it's passing off already—it's only a bruise. . . .
> They were all in good health. It could not be called ill health if Ivan Ilych sometimes said that he had a queer taste in his mouth and felt some discomfort in his left side. . . . The pain did not grow less, but Ivan Ilych made efforts to force himself to think that he was better. And he could do this so long as nothing agitated him. But as soon as he had any unpleasantness with his wife, and lack of success in his official work, or had bad cards at bridge, he was at once acutely sensible of his disease.

In previous research with cardiac patients (Levy, 1981), I analyzed this tendency to normalize symptoms of an incipient myocardial infarction throughout the early stages of an impending attack. Although cancer is for the most part an insidiously developing disease, and a heart attack is usually a dramatic event with an acute onset, this same human process of "typifying" and normalizing occurs in both instances. Excerpts from cardiac patient interviews dramatically demonstrate this human propensity to interpret disease symptoms in terms of the familiar, with sometimes lethal consequences related to treatment delay. Many of the patients expressed in fact a dogged sense of determination in their attempt to carry on as usual.

> I went out to the shop and worked for an hour and a half. One nitroglycerin pill was supposed to last four hours. For three days, I tried to work. Every day after dinner, I got this pain.

> As I was coming back, I got to feeling funny. I knew where I was, but it didn't seem like I was there. I pulled over [in the car] and began to feel better. I worked the rest of the evening.

> I'd sit in a chair for a couple of minutes and then go down and get some more logs. I got all the work done. . . . I'd work a few minutes and then have to quit [Levy, 1981, p. 160].

As Cowie (1976) and others have also found, virtually all of these cardiac patients attempted to *normalize* the early stages of an impending attack.

> Well, for four or five days before I came in, my chest was hurting. I thought I had eaten something. . . . Living alone, I don't eat normally.

> I began thinking it might be angina. [But] I had the same thing several years earlier, and then it was indigestion and gas [Levy, 1981, p. 160].

Unfortunately, this tendency to remain within the dominant, everyday reality until one is forced to alter the situational definition because of unavoidable biological sequellae (such as loss of breath or consciousness in a cardiac patient or severe weight loss or continuous rectal bleeding in a cancer patient) can be fatal.

Situational or mental factors also may be responsible for an individual's delay in securing a professional diagnosis of his symptoms. For example, an individual who is economically disadvantaged may be keenly aware of the abnormality of bodily symptoms, but other factors in daily living related to sheer survival simply take precedence over the diagnosis of an ailment. The following statement by an inner-city surgeon illustrates the situational difficulties faced by members of the lower socioeconomic class in just gaining access to health care:

> A third of the people admitted to surgery at ＿＿ Hospital in the year 1981 had no insurance at all. They were called "self-paid," which means no pay. So you have a woman who develops a lump. Her individual circumstances may include the point that she wonders about shelter, food, and she is trying to avoid crime in the community. These are all very significant personal problems. What are her options for having this lump examined, even if she decides it should be examined, which is the first stage? She doesn't have a private doctor. She will probably end up in an emergency room in a city hospital, such as ＿＿ . There, there will be other patients who appear to be sicker than she is, even if she is trying her best to go through this process. The others will take precedence. . . . And here we get into the behavior of doctors and the systems we ourselves have developed as medical people. She will be put to the back of the line. When she is seen, they may almost be saying "Why did you come here? There is really not much wrong with you. You should be going to the clinic." Then she will be referred to a clinic of some kind. Maybe it is a specialty clinic, maybe a surgery clinic, have another registration and waiting period. In fact, if she doesn't have a Medicaid card, she may be sent

downtown. This happens a lot, too. The point of
it is, if she gets through that process, unless special
things are done to eliminate the roadblocks that she
must face, she may perceive that the process of being diagnosed is more disturbing than the pain that
she has in her breast. She may then return to her
community, her home, the problems that she has to
face which she sees as immediate survival problems,
and the lump will grow [Freeman, 1982, n.p.].

Thus, individuals will ignore "obvious" symptoms—attributing
abdominal pains to indigestion, irregular or prolonged menses
to "stress," or irregular bowel activities to "the crazy diet I've
been on the last two months." Moreover, for at least some in
our society, and perhaps all of us to varying degrees, the mere
recognition that "something is not right" is not always sufficient to prompt the securing of adequate care. The subjective
appreciation of somatic symptoms, the motivation to present
oneself to proper medical expertise, and the means to do so—
all have to be considered as we examine the behavioral and social
factors contributing to adequate cancer management. In fact,
there are significant numbers of symptomatic persons who do
not enter the medical care system—or who enter too late. For
example, Hackett, Cassem, and Raker (1973) reported that over
40 percent of patients at an oncology clinic had waited four
months to one year or more before seeking care.

One would assume that individuals at high risk for disease
would be particularly vigilant in monitoring their physical status.
However, evidence suggests that this is not necessarily the case.
For example, incidence and mortality rates for breast and cervical cancer increase with age. Thirty-six percent of breast and
24 percent of cervical cancers occur in women over the age of
sixty-five. Forty-eight percent of deaths for breast cancer and
41 percent of mortality from cervical cancer also occur in this
age group. Yet Celentano, Shapiro, and Weisman (1982) found
that 23 percent of the elderly women in their community survey
had *never* had a Pap test, and 28 percent had not had one in
the previous five years. These elderly females were also signifi-

cantly less likely to report having breast examinations or performing breast self-examinations than younger interviewees.

Even more striking are the results from a second study, reported by Mulvihill, Safyer, and Bening (1982). These researchers examined the surveillance behavior of very high-risk women who were members of families genetically disposed toward breast cancer. While half the sample chose prophylactic mastectomy (having the breast removed before cancer had a chance to develop), the other half chose instead to forgo surgery and be monitored closely for symptoms. Their monitoring regimen included monthly practice of breast self-examination (BSE), baseline mammogram by twenty-five years of age, a repeat mammogram every two years till age forty, and yearly mammograms after that. At follow-up the investigators found that *none* of the individuals in the high-risk surveillance group were following the recommended regimen.

A number of investigators have studied the motivational factors associated with cancer detection behaviors (Schwoon and Schmoll, 1979; McCusker and Morrow, 1980; DiClemente and others, 1982). For example, McCusker and Morrow found that in a sample of middle-class professionals with easy access to the health care system, a prevention attitude on the part of the physician was crucial in motivating patients to participate in screening programs. In contrast, Schwoon and Schmoll's survey of blue-collar workers revealed that situational factors (finding spare time, obtaining baby sitters, and so on) played a major role in preventing participation in a cancer-screening program. Results from these two studies suggest that social class, with all its associated cultural and economic factors, needs to be taken into account in understanding the motivation underlying participation in cancer-screening programs.

In fact, Howard (1982a) has suggested that social class may differentially affect the detection of cancer at various sites. For example, cervical cancer detection (via Pap smears) may be avoided by the "hard-core," hard-to-reach disadvantaged, who remain for the most part outside the health care system. For middle-class American women, particularly the middle-aged and younger, the Pap test has become a routine way of life. But the situation is different for the early detection of breast cancer. Although late diagnosis of breast carcinoma is characteristic of some disadvantaged groups (for example, black females), lack of participation in breast cancer detection efforts is more uniformly spread across social classes than is true for cervical cancer screening. In fact, although women in low socioeconomic groups, black women, and multiparous women are more at risk for cervical cancer and have poorer ten-year survival rates, women in upper socioeconomic groups, white women, and childless or late primiparous women are most at risk for breast cancer. As Kegeles and Grady (1982) point out, such differential outcome by site of cancer may be in part influenced by various behavioral and social factors affecting participation in early-detection efforts.

Obviously, many factors—related to patient, physician, and health system variables—contribute to less than optimal health-monitoring behavior. In addition, some, if not most, of these factors interact with each other in affecting final health care delivery. For example, a financially disadvantaged person (patient variable) will likely wind up waiting interminably in a hospital clinic (system variable) and be seen intermittently by different (and sometimes indifferent) physicians (caregiver variable). All these negative factors combine to make continuous, good-quality medical care very unlikely.

Specific Screening and Early-Detection Technologies

For cancers in some sites, early detection is unlikely to affect eventual survival. For example, hepatic (liver) and pancreatic cancers are relatively rare but, once diagnosed, are rarely curable. "Catching" such tumors early would not at this stage of medical sciences contribute much in the way of survival advantage. On the other hand, the weight of the evidence suggests that survival rates for breast and cervical cancer are improved if these tumors are diagnosed at an early stage. In addition, early diagnosis and treatment of colorectal carcinoma and prostatic, testicular, and oral cancers may also enhance survival. Even in cases where early diagnosis and treatment do not appear to have overwhelming survival advantage, early treatment can have quality-of-life advantage in reducing morbidity associated with more radical treatment of advanced cases (Mettlin and Murphy, 1982).

As far as cancer-screening technology is concerned (that is, techniques appropriate for mass utilization in presumably healthy populations to detect cancer before it is clinically obvious), only the efficacy of mammography, plus physician breast palpation, has been demonstrated in a randomized clinical trial. The efficacy of the Pap test has been determined primarily by widespread and routine clinical use, coupled with the rather dramatic decline in mortality from uterine/cervical cancer associated with early detection and treatment of localized disease (Miller, 1982). For colon cancer, diagnostic techniques such as the use of sigmoidoscopy have proved effective; however, the efficacy of simpler and less costly tests, such as the fecal occult blood test to detect blood in the stools as an early sign of colon cancer, is still being evaluated (Winawer, 1980).

The World Health Organization (1981) has proposed that screening be limited to circumstances in which (1) the disease is a significant cause of morbidity and mortality, (2) the natural history is well understood, (3) there is a test that can detect the disease prior to the onset of signs and symptoms, (4) there is a specific treatment, (5) there is good evidence that early detection and treatment reduce morbidity and mortality, (6) expected benefits of early detection exceed risks and costs. Again, very few early-detection strategies satisfy all these requirements. Pap smears and breast palpation, plus mammography for women over fifty, are the only techniques that come close. In fact, the committee responsible for issuing this report cites cervical screening as the only technique that fulfills all the above criteria.

Early Detection of Breast Cancer. Periodic breast examinations by a physician; mammography, particularly for women over age fifty; and breast self-examination (BSE) are the three most commonly recommended early-detection strategies for breast cancer. The proportion of women polled who have had a physician-performed breast examination was 79 percent, as reported by Gallup in a 1980 survey of the public's awareness and use

of cancer detection tests. In that survey 43 percent of the women
respondents reported having been examined by a physician
within the past year. However, this survey, as well as other
surveys, also revealed that a smaller proportion had had repeat
examinations. For example, a survey of women's attitudes regarding breast cancer, conducted by Gallup in 1974, indicated
that 26 percent of the women surveyed had had fewer than five
examinations in the previous five years and that 24 percent had
had no examinations in the same period of time. Compared with
other groups in the surveys, those who reported fewer than five
examinations or no examinations tended to be older women,
women in low socioeconomic groups, and black women.

Parallel statistics exist for the practice of breast self-examination. Dramatic increases in public awareness regarding the
technique have occurred. Reported experience with BSE at least
once in a lifetime rose from 9 percent in the 1950s to 83 percent
in 1977. Again, however, only a small proportion of women
reported repeated practice of BSE, and only 18 percent reported
regular monthly practice (Kegeles and Grady, 1982).

Comparable figures on a national scale for the utilization
of mammography are available from the 1980 Gallup survey.
In that survey 59 percent of the women aged forty or over
reported never having had a mammogram; 14 percent of the
total sample reported having a mammogram every year, whereas
5 percent reported having mammograms less often than every
five years.

There is currently still some controversy over the recommended frequency by age category. Mammography was incorporated into a randomized clinical trial of breast cancer detection methods within the membership of the Health Insurance
Plan of Greater New York (referred to as the HIP study) (Shapiro, 1977). In this trial women (aged forty to sixty-four) were
randomly placed in one of two groups: a screened intervention
group and a group offered the usual care through the Health
Insurance Plan. Overall, there was a significant ten-year reduction in mortality of breast cancer for the screened group, but
this effect was limited to the older women (over age fifty).

Because of improved case finding by mammography since

this trial was completed, Miller (1982) has argued that perhaps mortality reduction would be found in younger women if the trial were conducted today. He also suggests that the reduction in mortality rates among the older women in the HIP study was attributable primarily to the physician's examination and not to the mammography by itself. Hence, mammography is not currently recommended for wide-scale public breast cancer screening. However, the American Cancer Society and the National Cancer Institute do recommend it for women over age fifty, despite the continuing controversy. Questions remain regarding the efficacy of combined mammography and breast palpation for younger women (aged forty to forty-five), as well as regarding the natural history of very small ("minimal") breast cancers discovered by mammography alone. Many of these minimal cancers may not be true malignancies and, if left alone, might not progress to full-blown carcinoma.

Nonetheless, mammography—coupled with careful, hands on palpation—can be an extremely useful clinical technique when administered by skilled technicians and clinicians, faced with a patient who has a suspicious symptom or complaint. The reduction in radiation dosage per mammogram has made it a relatively safe procedure. The effect of radiation in inducing breast cancer, in fact, is minimal in women over the age of thirty. Because mammography is not commonly recommended for mass public screening, however, it will not be considered further in this section. Rather, we will focus on the practice of BSE—its limits, as well as its efficacy, as a detection strategy—because it is wholly dependent on the behavior of the individual woman, our major interest here, and because much controversy has been generated around the practice of BSE in recent years.

The American Cancer Society recommends that BSE be performed monthly by all women over the age of twenty. However, according to Kegeles and Grady (1982), perhaps only 18–20 percent of the eligible female population habitually and regularly perform BSE, and even some of these women may not be performing it correctly. Most of the studies in this area rely on women's verbal self-report concerning their practice routine. In a review of the few existing studies that attempted to characterize *how* women were performing this self-examination, Holtzman and Celentano (1983, p. 1325) concluded that "each of the studies found that a substantial number of women who reported doing BSE did not know all the necessary steps."

Factors associated with the practice of BSE are age, education, and various attitudes and beliefs about cancer, its detection, and treatment potential. Although the literature is mixed in regard to these factors, in general the weight of the evidence suggests that older women, less educated women, and women who are anxious, have doubts about their ability to detect lumps accurately, and/or have a hopeless attitude about cancer treatment are less likely to perform BSE regularly. As noted earlier, epidemiological studies have generally indicated that middle-class, white, childless women are at greater risk for breast cancer, and since risk generally increases with age, the findings related to older women in the practice of BSE are perhaps the most significant.

But data from the Third National Cancer Survey (American Cancer Society, 1985) indicated that the incidence of breast cancer among black females has increased strikingly over the past four decades. In addition, studies have generally shown that black women who are diagnosed with breast cancer present with more advanced, and hence ultimately less curable, disease. Manfredi, Warneke, Graham, and Rosenthal (1977), in a survey of health behavior among black women, found that only 56 percent of the group of respondents most likely to benefit from BSE instruction—that is, those who perceived themselves at risk for breast cancer and believed in the benefit of early detection—knew about the technique of BSE or how to perform it.

Hard data providing the empirical basis on which the recommendation to practice BSE rests are rather scarce. The question of how much BSE contributes to reduced breast cancer mortality is currently very controversial. Advocates of BSE point out that the practice is cheap, always available, and has no inherent risks—except perhaps giving women either a false sense of security or, on the other hand, prompting unnecessary biopsies because of false finds. There is currently little evidence to substantiate either of these concerns. Who better than the woman herself can appreciate subtle internal, perceptual cues in change of tissue? Who would be more familiar with the usual breast texture, and hence most likely to detect the slightest change, than the woman herself? In fact, most breast cancers are discovered by the patient. Surely, therefore, it would be worthwhile to harness this self-perception and detection ability and to perfect it in a systematic fashion. At the least, BSE seems useful as an adjunct to a thorough medical examination.

On the other hand, there is currently no undisputable evidence that BSE by itself has any effect on breast cancer survival. As Howard (1984) points out, if those women who practice BSE are routinely receiving breast examinations by physicians, and mammography where appropriate, the additional contribution of BSE to early detection is probably minimal. More specifically, "BSE reduces mortality maybe [an additional] 5 or 10 percent if . . . its effect [is added to] mammography and physical exam. But alone, it may reduce mortality by 20 percent" (Howard, 1982b, p. 22).

The implications are therefore clear. Urging and teaching BSE as part of an individual prevention package seem to be appropriate. But major emphasis should be placed on recruiting high-risk women into health-screening programs and enhancing their compliance with follow-up referrals and recommendations. As Howard (1984) concludes, within the context of multimodality options for breast cancer control, BSE may be a beneficial component to each woman's main strategy, but it should not be advocated as a substitute modality. (For more extensive reviews of the BSE evidence, see Howard, 1984; Cole and Austin, 1981; Holtzman and Celentano, 1983.)

Early Detection of Cervical Cancer. There is less controversy about the usefulness of Pap tests in the early detection of cervical cancer and less dispute regarding populations that are yet underscreened and, hence, contain individuals who die needlessly. There is still some controversy, however, over frequency intervals and lifetime number of Pap tests per population screened (Miller, 1982).

In Canada and the United States, mortality from uterine/cervical cancer was decreasing before the widespread use of the

Pap test in screening programs. Such mortality reduction was likely due to changes in the prevalence of risk factors related to changing sexual practices between the two world wars and changes in overall improved medical care. In a series of Canadian studies, mortality rates before and after the implementation of cervical cancer–screening programs—including one that controlled for the effect of hysterectomy in the study population (using only "uteri at risk," rather than women at risk, for the analysis of mortality rates)—were compared. The results of these studies suggested that cervical and uterine mortality is reduced as a result of Pap test screening activity (Miller, 1982). On later analysis this association with screening intensity disappeared. Miller (1982, p. 44) therefore concluded that screening may make only a "limited contribution to the reduction of mortality and not be capable of abolishing mortality from the disease" (Miller, 1982, p. 44). He suggests a number of explanations for the change in trend, including the possibility that screening programs are concentrating on the wrong group of women; that is, they are not concentrating on the recruitment of high-risk women. It is also possible that there is now a rising incidence of cervical cancer in the population, because of changes in risk factors (for example, changes in sexual behavior patterns)—so that, if it were not for screening programs, there would be an epidemic of cervical cancer and indeed increased mortality from this disease.

    Miller (1982) suggests that, given the higher rates of carcinoma *in situ* that are diagnosed in younger women, more frequent tests should be performed in younger, rather than older, females. Wright and Riopelle (1982) have concluded that an early age of first intercourse, especially between the ages of fifteen and seventeen, is the most important epidemiological risk factor in the development of cervical cancer. They therefore urge that a Pap screening program based on numbers of years of sexual intercourse would be more efficient than one based on chronological age consideration. Such a cytological examination should be focused on the time period when most cases of cervical cancer develop: six to twenty years following first intercourse.

    As with the practice of BSE, Gallup surveys over the years

(on the public's awareness and use of cancer detection tests) indicate that women's knowledge of the Pap test has increased—from 77 percent in 1963 to 90 percent in 1970. These same surveys also indicate that increasing numbers of women have had at least one screening. Similarly, about 75 percent of the women polled in a National Center for Health Statistics (1975) survey had had at least one Pap test. However, fewer than one third of all women have repeat tests, and there are no figures available on how many women take tests at the intervals recommended by the American Cancer Society (yearly for women between eighteen and thirty-five years old and every five years for women over thirty-five) or the National Institutes of Health (every one to three years) (Kegeles and Grady, 1982).

Attitudinal studies have revealed similar factors associated with cervical screening as were found for breast cancer screening: fear of cancer, embarrassment regarding the test, and skepticism about the cure of cancer. A shift in some of these factors has been found to correspond with an increase in Pap smear utilization. Knopf (1976), studying changes in women's opinions about cancer over a seven-year period (1966–1973), found that at the later date more women reported a belief in cancer curability and endorsed the value of early detection, and this attitude shift was associated with increases in screening behavior.

Cost-benefit analyses of screening efficacy indicate that the most important screening test in a woman's lifetime is the first one. One test statistically results in a maximum return for the time and cost invested. Clearly, the most important aim, then, is to recruit women into screening programs for the first time—particularly high-risk, young, and sexually active women, as well as elderly and minority women who have not yet entered the screening system. Once a woman is in the system, a systematic and aggressive follow-up routine should be maintained. Although there is still controversy over the frequency and overall number of screens in a lifetime, repeat Pap tests are very important. Miller (1982) suggests the implementation of computerized, centralized registries in order to keep track of populations in a whole region and notify individuals for follow-up screens. Such a system may be more feasible for countries such as Great

Britain or Canada, where there is more central government control over medical practice. In the United States, where the private physician's office is the usual system unit, such a national
or regional screening communication network is less likely to
develop.

*Early Detection of Colorectal, Prostate, Testicular, and Oral Can-
cers.* Colorectal, prostate, testicular, and oral cancer sites are
reasonably accessible by looking and feeling; therefore, early
detection is at least possible. The rate of testicular cancer for
males peaks in young adulthood, and the disease is most common in late adolescence and in the twenty-to-thirty age range.
Although there have never been the public campaigns to promote testicular self-examination as there have been for BSE,
young males should be taught to self-examine for changes in
testicular character, such as the presence of a nontender mass
that might be indicative of malignant change.

Early detection of prostatic cancer—which has increasing incidence with age and is most common in elderly males—
is most efficiently accomplished by digital rectal examination
by a physician (Guinan and others, 1981). As Guinan and colleagues point out, the digital examination is universally available
(if individuals have access to a physician), because physicians
tend to include it routinely as part of any physical examination
of a male—especially for men over forty. The digital examination provides directly useful information about the rectum and
anal sphincter, and "in this age of escalating medical costs and
physician accountability for these costs, you can't beat the cost
of a digital rectal examination" (p. 145).

Oral cancer accounts for approximately 5-6 percent of
all cancers in the United States and causes approximately 7,000
deaths a year. And yet this form of malignancy is rather easily
accessible for early detection, affording the opportunity for early
diagnosis and less aggressive, radical treatment. The most common site for cancer of the oral cavity is the lip, especially the
lower lip, followed by the tongue, floor of the mouth, gingiva,
buccal mucosa, and palate. Innocent-appearing irritations, small
changes in the epithelial structure, and changes in color and
swellings can be signs of potential oral cancer. Epidemiologically

identified individuals most at risk for cancer at this site include persons with a history of tobacco use, heavy alcohol consumption, and poor oral hygiene. Oral cancer is found more frequently in males, and incidence rises with age.

Many of the deaths that result from this malignancy, unfortunately, are at least in part due to late detection and, hence, advanced disease at diagnosis. Dentists should be trained in cancer screening and taught to educate their patients about good hygiene and early cancer symptoms, so that every dentist's office becomes a locus for cancer control. Unfortunately, even if that ideal state were to exist, there would still be unmonitored groups in this country because they lack access to dental care.

Finally, the high incidence of colorectal cancer in the United States—138,000 cases a year—justifies a major screening effort. The rectosigmoid area of the colon can be examined by rigid or flexible sigmoidoscopy. The latter is better tolerated by patients but is used by only a limited number of specialists in this country. The rigid sigmoidoscope has never been popular with either patients or physicians and is not deemed feasible for wide-scale screening. The remainder of the colon beyond the sigmoid area can be examined by fecal occult blood testing, X ray, and endoscopy.

As in all of our discussion in this chapter, it is important to distinguish between diagnostic and screening tests. The barium enema, used in conjunction with colonoscopy, has greatly enhanced the detection of early colon cancer. Because of the time, expense, and minimal but nevertheless increased risks involved, however, such a technique could not be used for screening presumably healthy individuals, except those who fall into a high-risk category (for example, those with a family history of polyposis, or those who have had chronic ulcerative colitis for longer than seven years,or those with a past history of female genital cancer).

As a screening device, the fecal occult blood test certainly requires more patient participation in the examination process than the sigmoidoscope does. While the sigmoidoscope examination is more expensive and requires the patient to schedule an appointment with a physician, the currently used fecal occult blood test (the Hemoccult, or HO) requires a rather elaborate behavioral compliance sequence. The individual taking the test is instructed to prepare "six smears, during three days, from different parts of stool specimens while on a high-fiber, meat-free diet, with abstinence of vitamins, aspirin-containing compounds, and large amounts of peroxidase-containing vegetables" (Winawer, 1980, p. 1095). Because the test is not specific for human hemoglobin, or even for hemoglobin in general, it does have a reported false-positive rate of between .5 percent and 2.1 percent. As Winawer points out, any false positive is unacceptable in a mass screening program, since it results in unnecessary, invasive, diagnostic procedures for those individuals who do not have cancer.

Before screening tests—including the HO—can be systematically evaluated in a randomized fashion in order to demonstrate genuine survival value for those diagnosed early as a result of screening, individuals in evaluation studies need to comply with the test's requirements; and appropriate persons need to be recruited into the study—especially high-risk individuals— so that relatively large numbers of cases would be detected through screening and follow-up. Therefore, it is important to understand reasons for participation or nonparticipation, as well as the factors related to compliance with screening requirements. And because the fecal occult blood test is a patient-centered technology, requiring skilled participation and compliance on the part of the person, it will be our focus here.

Two recent studies (Dent, Bartrop, Goulston, and Chapuis, 1983; Morrow, Way, Hoagland, and Cooper, 1982) showed that, in general, individuals whose regular physicians are themselves prevention oriented are more likely to participate and follow through with slide preparation and return. Noncompliers are more likely to be elderly or to be indifferent to the value of health checks and screening tests. Winawer (1980) notes that—in contrast to compliance for screening with sigmoidoscopy, which has always been low—compliance for fecal occult blood tests is generally high in controlled studies using well-motivated participants (in both of the studies cited above, participation rates were approximately 40 percent of those approached); but compliance is much lower among the general public when no prior educational program has been instituted.

Our knowledge in this area is still rudimentary. We have few definitive data regarding mortality reduction efficacy for colorectal tests, including optimal frequency of screens for high-risk populations; and we are only beginning to examine the adequacy of patient-centered tests, such as BSE and the Hemoccult test, as well as motives, attitudes, and related knowledge in population subgroups at risk.

Effects of Delay in Diagnosis of Suspicious Symptoms

Concern over the question of diagnostic delay is a long-standing one. Wainwright (1911) focused on clinical problems associated with patient delay, and Pack and Gallo (1938) arbitrarily defined a delayed diagnosis as any diagnosis of a suspicious cancer symptom made three or more months after the symptom was first noticed. Antonovsky and Hartman (1974), reviewing all the studies between 1938 and 1969 that used this three-month delay criterion, found that 44 percent of the patients in these studies belonged in the "delay" group. In our own study with breast cancer patients at the National Institutes of Health, approximately 25 percent delayed seeking a diagnosis of their malignancy for three months or longer.

Beyond simply calculating the extent of delay in various patient subgroups, a number of studies have also attempted to estimate the impact of delay time on prognosis and survival (Worden and Weisman, 1975; Wilkinson and others, 1979; Bosl and others, 1981; Elwood and Moorehead, 1980; Gould-Martin and others, 1982; DiClemente and others, 1982). Elwood and Moorehead examined records of approximately 1,500 females with breast cancer and found that delay in diagnosis increased the chances of cancer's being diagnosed at a later stage of disease and also decreased five-year survival. In another study of the impact of both physician and patient delay on testicular cancer stage at diagnosis, Bosl and associates (1981) reported that the joint delay of patients and physicians was directly related to clinical stage of cancer at diagnosis: "The median patient plus physician delay for stage I was 75 days; for stage II, 102 days; and for stage III, 134 days ($\underline{p}$ < 0.017)'' (p. 970). In contrast, some investigators report no relationship between delay and cancer outcome (Fisher, Redmond, and Fisher, 1977; Dennis, Gardner, and Lim, 1975). However, because of selection biases, interpretation of such findings should be considered with caution (Eddy and Eddy, 1984).

The whole question of delay is a very complex one. First, methodologically, data on delay time are typically collected retrospectively; that is, the investigators rely on patients' reports of how long they were aware of the symptom's existence before acting. Obviously, a number of factors can affect estimates of delay time, including underestimation of delay because of perceived personal responsibility and guilt experienced when cancer is finally diagnosed. Such an underestimate would then bias the study's results by making it appear that the delay time did not have serious consequences for stage of diagnosis or survival. Other measurement issues also tend to obscure the effects of delay on cancer outcome. Studies that focus on stage of diagnosis as the outcome variable related to delay are possibly focusing on too crude a biological end-point measure to be useful in evaluating the effects of delay behavior. For example, one individual diagnosed as ''stage I, breast cancer'' may have small, but invasive, tumor cell foci; another may have more extensive, but still localized, tumor masses. Within this same stage, then, differential effects of delay time can still be operative. Only when survival is the end point can the true appreciation of the delay effects be determined.

The effects of delay can also be overestimated if what is referred to as ''lead-time'' bias is not controlled. If person A notices barely perceptible breast cancer symptoms and immediately comes in for a diagnosis, her survival time may be calculated from date of diagnosis. If person B ignores obvious symptoms, and comes in for diagnosis at a relatively advanced stage, her survival time will also be counted from date of diagnosis to date of death. By these measures person A probably will have a much longer survival time, calculated in months, than person B. However, person A's clock time for calculating purposes may have been simply shifted backward (she just knew longer that she had cancer), but there may have been little actual survival advantage to early detection. This lead-time bias can be adjusted for in survival analyses, and—as Eddy and Eddy (1984) point out—in any case would possibly not have much of a biasing effect, since delay is usually a matter of months at most.

In addition, the actual biology of the tumor needs to be taken into account in any consideration of the effects of delay. Pater, Loeb, and Siu (1979) reported the poorest prognosis in those patients who had the *shortest* delay interval coupled with a change in tumor symptom during that period. In all likelihood, the most aggressive tumors change rapidly, and even a short delay interval will not contribute much to survival in these cases.

In a discussion of methodological biases in studies of the effect of delay on cancer outcome, Eddy and Eddy (1984, p. 36) conclude that the net effect of such biases has probably been to underestimate the impact of delay on cancer treatment outcome: "While it is not possible to make definitive statements, it appears that when patients who do not delay are compared with those who delay more than three months, there is a decrease in long-term survival on the order of 10–20 percent. If true, this is a sizable reduction in survival."

Assuming, then, that delay in reporting to a physician for a diagnosis of a suspicious cancer symptom is a serious and significant contributor to poor cancer prognosis for at least some cancer sites, then it becomes a matter of grave importance to know who does not behave in a health-appropriate fashion, and why. Again, the literature in this regard is not very enlightening. Demographically, older, poorer, and less educated individuals tend to come in for diagnosis with already advanced disease. Those who are not connected to a health delivery system, or who are community isolates, and those who are psychologically depressed or otherwise emotionally disturbed also have been reported to delay in obtaining diagnosis (Eddy and Eddy, 1984). As mentioned earlier, among the reasons offered by patients to account for delay are financial cost, fear of cancer, failure to appreciate the value of prompt diagnosis and early treatment, inconvenience, and embarrassment over the examination pro-

cess. No attempt has been made to weigh the relative importance of such factors in specific population subgroups or for
various tumor site diagnosis.

   Using such reported factors as a basis for analysis, Eddy
and Eddy (1984) developed a clever decision matrix based on
subjective cost-benefit assessment on the part of the patient, in
order to understand why one individual would be prompted to
report for early cancer detection and another individual would
not. Earlier in this chapter, an inner-city surgeon's description
of a typical patient seen in a public clinic was quoted. The
woman referred to weighed the cost of reporting downtown for
a proper card and returning to another clinic for another in-
definite wait; and she decided that the costs for *her* outweighed
the benefit of diagnosis and treatment, if warranted. So she went
home, and the lump grew. If the lump was malignant, however,
this was not the most "rational" decision, because eventually
she will be biologically overwhelmed by the cancer, will be
diagnosed and treated with advanced disease, will suffer great
pain and discomfort as a result of radical treatment, and will
likely die relatively soon after treatment initiation due to widely
disseminated malignancy. If she had known what her odds were
of actually having cancer, based on her particular symptoms
and overall risk factors; if she had understood the odds of successful treatment, assuming that cancer was diagnosed at that
point; and if she could have weighed the actual value of inconvenience and uncertainty until the diagnosis was made, she would
have been able to make an eminently rational choice. However,
as Eddy and Eddy point out, few people—even physicians—
can accurately access the actual possibility of cancer, taking into
account all known risk factors that apply in a particular case.
Even if those numbers are known, irrational factors—such as
denial or an overestimate of inconvenience and cost—come into
play, often prompting delay. From a public health perspective,
and on the basis of the evidence that delay has a negative prognostic impact, Eddy and Eddy estimate that 10,000 to 50,000
new cases of cancer each year could be cured if delay could be
eliminated. In addition, many thousand person-years of life
could be gained for patients each year. In the balance is the

relatively low cost of diagnosis and treatment—particularly compared to treatment of other chronic diseases, such as hypertension. The task, then, is to educate the public as much as possible about the relative significance of various symptoms and about the potential for cure through early treatment. Perhaps an explicit "walking through" of the pros and cons of seeking early diagnosis could be attempted in order to help people better understand the benefits of early care.

Role of Physicians and Health Care Agencies in Promoting Early Detection

Most of the factors that affect health delivery have to do with the delivery process itself—physician and system characteristics that enhance or provide obstacles to early cancer care. Physicians who are prevention oriented enhance the probability that their patients will also be conscious of good health behavior, including cancer-screening practices, and will participate in screening opportunities when provided. And there is abundant evidence that physician characteristics summed up as a good "bedside manner," including continuity in the patient-physician relationship, enhance health care delivery.

We have not considered the whole issue of insurance reimbursement for routine screening checks. Insurance claims usually are tied to diagnosis of potential disorders. Consequently, there are financial, as well as time, constraints on physician's willingness to make every office a screening program site. Either the patients must bear the cost burden of the procedure, or physicians must say that they are looking for something suspicious, even if they are not. Physicians also are unwilling to spend expensive office time and effort on screening activities with little financial payoff. But, as Fox (1981) points out, physicians are also teachers. In addition to teaching patients the techniques of self-examination and the proper appreciation of symptom significance, they are teachers of other fledgling physicians and have the opportunity to demonstrate, by word as well as deed, the practice of preventive medicine related to early cancer detection.

Systems variables that enhance health care delivery by

affecting a patient's willingness to participate in screening and detection activities include physical access to facilities, office hour and clinic wait time, and financial cost. Agencies can encourage participation in such programs by providing transportation to health care facilities, baby-sitting services on premises, evening and Saturday office hours, sliding fees for services, and minimal wait time while in the clinic.

Health care agencies, including the federal government, also should attempt to educate the public in a more sophisticated understanding of what is meant by elevated risk on an individual basis. If a woman has a threefold elevated risk of developing breast cancer because she has a history of chronic fibrocystic disease, what does this mean for Mrs. A., who has such a history and is also childless and has a sister and an aunt who have had breast cancer? Physicians need to understand the epidemiological data related to risk status, and they need to be able to impart such information in a manner that is not too frightening. And, as discussed earlier, more general information could be made available regarding the probability of malignancy, given certain symptoms in particular population subgroups. For example, as Eddy and Eddy (1984) point out, in an individual with one of the warning signs publicized by the American Cancer Society, there is a greater than 1-in-100 chance that malignancy will be diagnosed. A person who experiences prolonged or unusual vaginal or rectal bleeding will know, then, that the chances of actually having cancer are better than 1 percent. Such knowledge, based on empirical data, provides the possibility of a rational weighing of cost (tangible and intangible) against the diagnostic odds.

Such an effort to inform the public of relative risks and the weighting of symptom significance has never been carried out, and it is unclear how such a rational approach would interact with cultural, social, and individual personality variables in affecting cancer detection behavior. But it is an important public health question and needs to be examined in a systematic way, perhaps through a pilot effort that could then be evaluated for effectiveness in altering the behavior of population subgroups—particularly those at actual highest risk.

Compliance with Therapeutic Regimens

From the time of his visit to the doctor, Ivan Ilych's chief occupation was the exact fulfillment of the doctor's instructions regarding hygiene and the taking of medicine, and the observation of his pain and his excretions. His chief interests came to be people's ailments and people's health. When sickness, disease, or recoveries were mentioned in his presence, especially when the illness resembled his own, he listened with agitation which he tried to hide, asked questions, and applied what he heard to his own case. . . . His wife had adopted a definite line in regard to his illness and kept to it regardless of anything he said or did. Her attitude was this. "You know," she would say to her friends, "Ivan Ilych can do as other people do, and keep the treatment prescribed for him. One day, he'll take his drops and keep strictly to his diet and go to bed in good time, but the next day, unless I watch him, he'll suddenly forget his medicine, eat sturgeon—which is forbidden—and sit up playing cards till one o'clock in the morning."

"Oh, come, when was that?" Ivan Ilych would ask in vexation. "Only once at Peter Ivanovitch's."

"And yesterday, with Shebek."

"Well, even if I hadn't stayed up, this pain would have kept me awake."

"Be that as it may, you'll never get well like that, but will always make us wretched" [Tolstoy, (1886) 1960, pp. 120, 123, 125].

Despite Ivan Ilych's intense preoccupation with his increasing pain, he still deviates from prescription—in part because he deems the regimen ineffective and ultimately useless. As we shall see, compliance or noncompliance with medical regimens is a complex affair. And underlying factors undoubtedly shift depending on developmental stage. Noncompliance in a young pediatric oncology patient has a different significance from noncompliance in an older adolescent or an eighty-year-old widower. Physicians can also choose to deviate from prescribed regimens. We shall explore some of these complexities in this section.

Extent of and Reasons for Patient Noncompliance. The points that were raised regarding physician and system variables associated with patient participation in screening programs can also be made in regard to patient compliance with treatment regimens. There is certainly no sharp demarcation in the health care delivery system between early detection, diagnosis, and treatment of cancer. The process is a continuum of patient-physician-system interaction.

Although treatment compliance is an extensive area of research in its own right (Haynes, Taylor, and Sackett, 1979), relatively little research has been carried out specifically with cancer patients. One of the first published studies in the area of cancer patient noncompliance was conducted with pediatric cancer patients (Smith, Rosen, Trueworthy, and Lowman, 1979). The investigators found that 33 percent of the pediatric leukemia and lymphoma patients studied did not comply with their prescribed oral prednisone regimen. And when they stratified by age, they found that 59 percent of the older adolescents did not comply with the prescription. One major reason that adolescents do not comply with selected drug regimens is that such agents cause embarrassing, and socially disruptive, side effects. Adolescents are acutely sensitive about their appearance, and drugs that cause weight gain, hair loss, or skin eruptions are particularly unlikely to be taken according to prescription. The following case is illustrative:

> The patient was a black male who was diagnosed at age thirteen as having acute lymphoblastic leukemia in May 1975. The family (parents, patient, one sibling) was stable and fit into the Hollingshead and Redlich Class II (upper middle class). The patient and his parents were told the diagnosis and prognosis, and considerable time was spent in an-

swering their questions. The patient and his mother attended educational sessions about the disease as well as group sessions dealing with living with the disease, which were part of an active program of social support. The father lived in the home but would not accompany his son on clinical appointments nor visit him when he was hospitalized.

Initial treatment consisted of vincristine and prednisone, and maintenance therapy consisted of daily 6-mercaptopurine, weekly methotrexate, and a course of prednisone every fourth month. This patient had no medically severe side effects during induction or maintenance, but he was distressed by the body changes associated with therapy (for example, hair loss, weight gain, facial puffiness).

In late April 1977, the patient experienced a bone marrow relapse. The physician set up a meeting with the patient and his parents to discuss the significance of the disease with relapse. During this meeting, the patient admitted that he had taken his medicines only intermittently during the recent months. It was again explained to the patient that the disease control depended upon a full dose of medicine and that without the medicine the disease would progress and the patient could die. The patient was then treated as an outpatient with vincristine and prednisone. At the end of the twenty-eight days, the bone marrow was still in relapse and the 17 kgs [ketogenic steroids in urine] assay indicated prednisone noncompliance. . . .

The patient was then admitted to the hospital and treated with prednisone, vincristine, and L-asparaginase. A bone marrow aspirate three weeks later showed that a remission had been achieved. At this time (6/23/77), the repeat urine assay showed that the patient was compliant in taking his prednisone [Smith, Cairns, Sturgeon, and Lansky, 1981, p. 297].

We know from the general compliance literature that chronicity and complexity of regimen are associated with poor drug compliance. As cancer therapy has become more effective and patients remain alive longer, it is likely that chronic, oral, self-administered maintenance regimens will become more and more commonplace. Because of this likelihood, understanding factors associated with cancer patient noncompliance is of paramount importance.

A major difficulty in conducting studies in this area concerns the availability of valid and reliable measurements of compliant behavior. Valid assays have been developed for detecting blood levels or traces of drug metabolites for a few common anticancer drugs. Smith, Rosen, Trueworthy, and Lowman (1979) utilized an assay measuring urinary 17-ketogenic steroids (17 kgs) as a reflection of prednisone ingestion. Although they argue that this assay is a valid and reliable one, others (Lilleyman, French, and Young, 1981) have questioned its validity as a marker of drug compliance. Levels of 17 kgs can be greatly influenced by individual differences in absorption rates and, hence, the bioavailability of the drug. In addition to direct measures of patient compliance such as blood drug levels, and objective counts of gross compliance indicators, such as appointment keeping, indirect methods of measurement—such as pill counts and patient self-report of medication adherence—are frequently used. Although early research suggested that patients tended to overreport compliance with drug taking (Gordis, Markowitz, and Lillienfeld, 1969), more recent work suggests that there is a fairly high positive correlation between patients' reports of medication taking and certain biological indications of medication adherence (Green, Levine, and Deeds, 1975). Therefore, until valid, efficient, and reasonably inexpensive assays are developed, perhaps patients can be taught to monitor and validly report their own drug-taking behavior.

Our focus has been on drug compliance because at least some orally administered chemotherapy agents are self-administered, and the opportunity for noncompliance is both great and difficult to monitor. Of course, compliance involves more than drug taking on the part of patients. Patients also may not

adhere to surgical and radiation treatments or to ancillary requirements—such as dental hygienic and preventive treatments
in patients undergoing head and neck radiation—aimed at the
prevention of morbidity.

Because little systematic research has been conducted on
cancer patient compliance, there are few data available regarding the actual extent of the problem. In major research centers,
where patient-to-staff ratio is very good and patients are particularly motivated to become part of the team effort, noncompliance—particularly with in-house treatments—may be relatively infrequent. Practicing community oncologists tend to
report more difficulties with patient cooperation and view the
issue of noncompliance as a rather serious one. But as least one
report (Hoagland, Morrow, Bennett, and Carnrike, 1983) suggests the opposite—namely, that physicians conducting experimental clinical trials may have more problems with compliance
than community physicians do. According to Hoagland and
associates, research physicians—in seeking the informed consent of participants in the trials—are required to admit that they
do not know whether the experimental treatment will prove to
be more effective than the standard treatment. Such an admission may undermine the patient's confidence and enhance the
likelihood of noncompliance.

In addition, despite increasingly effective therapies, an
unacceptably large number of patients still fail to improve.
Many, if not most, of such failures can be accounted for on the
basis of tumor biology (for example, resistance of tumor to particular treatment regimens or aggressive metastatic spread of
neoplastic cells); but if even a portion of such failures can be attributed to the lack of patient or physician compliance, then such
failures can be potentially prevented. There is evidence, for instance, that failure to take the full dose requirements of anticancer drugs is associated with increased treatment failure rates.
Bonadonna and Valagussa (1981) found that elderly women
did as well as younger women under treatment for breast cancer—if they took the full treatment dose despite toxicity. Although the general compliance literature suggests that toxic side
effects are not strongly associated with noncompliance, side

effects may induce some patients to drop out of treatment. For example, Lazlo, Lucas, and Huang (1981) noted that approximately half of their patients with disseminated testicular cancer missed appointments or delayed the course of toxic cis-platinum, vinblastine, and bleomycin treatment because of severe nausea and vomiting. Smith, Rosen, Trueworthy, and Lowman (1979), in their study of adolescent noncompliance, also found that noncompliance rates in the older children were affected by treatment side effects—weight gain and skin changes. Such side effects are particularly troublesome to adolescents, who are already painfully aware of body changes and have strong social approval needs.

Active Noncompliance: Unorthodox Treatments. Although humans have always tended to self-medicate, outside of or along with traditional medical care, in recent years the issue of "alternative cancer therapies" has come to public attention by media coverage of the Laetrile controversy and vitamin cancer treatment of such notables as the actor Steve McQueen. Historically, unorthodox treatments for malignancy have ranged from devices such as the orgone energy device—a zinc-lined box in which the patient reposed while receiving cosmic energy—to grape diets and massive doses of vitamin C (Henney, 1982).

There has been very little in the way of systematic research regarding who uses alternative forms of cancer therapy and why, as well as what effects such treatments have on cancer morbidity and mortality in the United States. Other than the well-publicized clinical trial of Laetrile efficacy (Moertel and others, 1982), and the earlier investigations of the Hoxsey treatment (consisting of "pink medicine"—lactated pepsin and potassium iodine—and "black medicine"—cascara in prickly ash bark and other vegetation) and Krebiozen by the federal government during the 1950s and 1960s, scientific studies of such agents have not been carried out. Recent work by Cassileth (1982) and Pendergrass and Davis (1981) has begun to shed some light on the proportion of adults and pediatric patients "at risk" for use of unorthodox treatment. In a survey of adult cancer patients, Cassileth reports that 78 percent of patients in standard treatment had at least heard of alternative treatments and that 10 percent of those patients admitted that they had received or were currently receiving unorthodox therapies. Pendergrass and Davis found that parents who expressed desperation about their child's condition, who were dissatisfied with their role in the child's treatment, or who were looking for "an easier treatment method" were at greatest risk for seeking unorthodox therapies.

Cassileth has raised an interesting point about the current unorthodox treatments. Historically, she notes, cancer patients have always resorted to self-medications, but in the past these treatments assumed the form of drugs or various devices. And, although such "treatments" were rarely scientifically tested, they *could be* evaluated by rigorous empirical examination, with the potential for banishment from the market and, hence, publicly controlled. However, in this post-Laetrile era, the currently thriving unorthodox treatments involve life-style changes and spiritual "mind control": clean living, pure diet, and spiritual exercises. Such treatments are not amenable to any form of empirical examination and hence are virtually impossible to disprove.

This whole movement related to thought and body control is part of a larger self-help zeitgeist that has been growing in popularity since the 1970s. "Patient-centric technologies" (Levy and Howard, 1982) endow the patients themselves with a sense of competency and control over their health and destiny. Healthy people, as well as those who are chronically ill, are learning to diagnose, monitor, and treat their own symptoms, and only selectively call for professional help when their lay expertise needs assistance. Even the practice of breast self-examination can be viewed as one technique within the armamentarium of the self-care feminist movement. "These women are formulating ideologies and tactics that protect their lay-oriented technologies from professional dominance and co-option. Their right to practice and use the hardware of the medical establishment (for example, the speculum) has been challenged, but their softer techniques involving education and indoctrination may be less susceptible to professional scrutiny and control" (Levy and Howard, 1982, p. 575).

On the one hand, there is clear danger in such lay co-opting of medical care specialization. Unproven treatments are substituted for standard therapies, and lives are potentially lost in the process. On the other hand, there are "patient-centric technologies" that rightfully reside within the lay domain. Such expertise includes the perception and reporting of symptoms, self-monitoring of physical status, and the sharing of knowledge and the process of informed consent. As Cassileth (1982) concludes, although we may not wish to recommend wheat grass therapy—or any of the other myriad alternative treatments for cancer, from snake meat to olive oil—we might want to consider the patient's need for some sense of control and self-determination in the treatment process. Particularly with a disease as erratic as cancer, the need may be all the greater for patients to be involved in their own care.

Patient-Physician Relationship and Physician Noncompliance. It is certainly inappropriate to focus on patient behavior alone. As we saw in the section on screening and early detection, a potent factor affecting extent of cooperation is the nature of the patient-physician relationship, with all the intangibles that that implies. Competence, communication ease, continuity of relationship, interest on the part of the physician, and many other facets of the relationship play a part in enhancing or inhibiting the patient's cooperative participation in the treatment process. Again, there has been very little research directly related to cancer patients and their treating oncologists. "The relationship between active participation by the cancer patient in medical/surgical decision making and subsequent compliance deserves careful evaluation, as does the effect on compliance of the physician's commitment to the therapeutic regimen and willingness to support the patient both emotionally and physically during a period of adverse reaction" (Lewis, Linet, and Abeloff, 1983, p. 676).

Apart from patient behavior, and the patient-physician relationship associated with compliance rates in cancer patients, the physician himself supplies a source of variance in treatment compliance. Physician underprescribing, deviating from standard treatment, and departing from experimental protocol treatments on the basis of extraneous judgmental factors (such as patient age or socioeconomic level) are relatively unexplored areas in the cancer field. And such deviations, if they occur, clearly invalidate the experiments. For a valid and clinically useful therapeutic trial outcome, a numerically adequate sample of eligible patients must be randomized into the trial in a timely fashion. In addition, if the trial outcome is ultimately to be clinically useful, then the study results must be generalizable to the appropriate target clinical population at large. If the sample of trial participants is biased in some unknown fashion, then no matter how scientifically sound the trial concept and design, and statistically clean the results, the outcome is clinically useless for all *practical* purposes.

Anecdotal evidence, as well as recent study data (Taylor, Margolese, and Soskolne, 1984; McCusker, Wax, and Bennett, 1982; Lee, Marks, and Simpson, 1980), suggests that these two major principles of trial conduct may in fact be frequently violated. A sizable number of trials have closed because—as a result of competition with other protocols, undue toxicity of the experimental agent, the departure of the principal investigator, staff apathy, or oncologists' refusals to refer eligible patients—no more participants could be found. And, as McCusker, Wax, and Bennett (1982) have demonstrated, trial samples have been biased by late referrals of study patients after all other possible treatments had been tried and by the elimination of eligible patients from low socioeconomic groups (presumably because of a physician's private judgments regarding the noncompliance of such individuls). As a result, many patients were sicker than expected before they participated in the study trial, so that the new treatment could not be adequately tested; and, since there are probably real host differences between socioeconomic levels (Berg, Ross, and Latourette, 1977), generalizability from the trial results was jeopardized. In all these instances, the trial process was clearly affected by physicians' decisions and behavior. Systematic research in this area is needed in order to increase the effectiveness of clinical trials and to change physicians' attitudes associated with trial conduct. The aim of such behavior change would be an increase in timely referrals and a more adequate sampling of patients representative of appropriate patient populations at large.

Informed Consent in Trials. Federal regulations concerning the protection of human subjects require that patients selected for biomedical research must be informed specifically about procedures, purposes, risks and benefits, and alternative options; of their right to terminate experimental treatment without prejudice; and of their right to question staff regarding treatment procedures (45 *Code of Federal Regulations* 46 (1978)). They must also be advised whether monetary compensation will be provided if injuries occur during the research project. Consent to treatment must be given voluntarily, without undue inducement or force, duress, fraud, constraint, or coercion. Presumably, a well-informed patient becomes less vulnerable to such deceit or coercion. In spite of these requirements, studies by Cassileth, Zupkis, Sutton-Smith, and March (1980) and by Grundner (1980) suggest that patients do not fully understand what they are told or what they read on consent forms. Typically, these forms—because of their technical, medical, and legal language—are comprehensible only to those whose reading ability is at the advanced college or graduate level. Consequently, truly *informed* consent is probably rare.

Knowledge, of course, does not guarantee free choice. Free and dispassionate choice is also more likely if the patient is not crippled by fear, depression, and distress. Ideally, the concept of informed consent is a mandate for patient self-determination. "The traditional paternalistic role of health practitioners is being defined as illegal and amoral if it perpetuates a monopoly of knowledge and stifles patients' independence. Under certain conditions, health providers may know better than patients what is in the patient's best interest—what 'gamble' he or she should elect. But modern rules and regulations forbid health professionals to implement their insight, benevolence, and good intention by convincing the patient of the wisdom of their perspective. Trust in the physician is not an acceptable substitute for informed consent" (Levy and Howard, 1982, p. 571). When a patient is clearly comatose or otherwise mentally incapacitated, others may act in his or her behalf. But short of that, the requirements for consent may be exacted when the patient is still not capable of fully rational behavior.

For example, Smith (1974) analyzed the consent process

during an emergency cardiac catheterization procedure. Because the patients were adults and conscious, the law required that they—and not someone acting on their behalf—be informed of the process and consent to it. However, because of the distress of the moment, most such patients could be classified as situationally mentally incompetent. Nevertheless, "consent" was obtained, although the informative process that ensued made a mockery of the law. Smith proposes that, under such circumstances, reasonable care on the part of the physician, assuming sole responsibility for the welfare of the patient, would fulfill the clinician's responsiblity in such a situation. "The formal requirement of [patient] consent, on the other hand, may allow precisely what the physician is normally not allowed to do: stifle the spirit of the law by observing it to the letter" (p. 403).

Despite the ideal to be striven for, rational and dispassionate choice cannot be extracted from desperate and anxious patients who cling to their physician and his or her treatment offering as the last hope for life. (For further discussion of these informed consent issues, see Lidz and others, 1984; Gray, 1975; Fletcher, Branson, and Freireich, 1979.) In fact, at some point on the treatment continuum, a fully sentient patient may view this "last hope for life" as no longer a reasonable expectancy. At that point, the issue of informed consent for treatment slides over into the right to forgo treatment in order to hasten the process of dying that is already under way. Although such a choice may be considered "noncompliance" to treatment in the strictest sense, most would view such a stance as a matter of individual choice and right to self-determination on the part of the patient.

"Noncompliance" in the Terminally Ill. In the following lengthy but poignant passage, Tolstoy ([1866] 1960, pp. 129–130, 137) conveys in Ivan Ilych's subjective musings the dawning self-awareness that one's own life is ending. He also captures the social withdrawal of others, which frequently accompanies the dying process, and the dying person's further alienation and isolation as a result of the pretense and denial of others.

"It's not a question of appendix or kidney trauma, but of life and death. Yes, life was there and now it is going, going, and I cannot stop it.

Yes. Why deceive myself? Isn't it obvious to every-
one but me that I'm dying, and that it's only a question of weeks, days. It may happen this moment.
There was light and now there is darkness. I was
here and now I am going there! Where?'' A chill
came over him, his grieving ceased, and he felt only
the throbbing of his heart.

"When I am not, what will there be? There
will be nothing. Then where shall I be when I am
no more? Can this be dying? No, I don't want to!"
He jumped up and tried to light the candle, felt
for it with trembling hands, dropped candle and
candlestick on the floor, and fell back on his pillow.

"What's the use? It makes no difference,"
he said to himself, staring with wide-open eyes into
the darkness. "Death. Yes, death. And none of
them know or wish to know it, and they have no
pity for me. Now they are playing." He heard
through the door the distant sound of a song and
its accompaniment. "It's all the same to them, but
they will die too! Fools! I first, and they later, but
it will be the same for them. And now they are
merry. The beasts!"

. . . What tormented Ivan Ilych most was the
deception, the lie, which for some reason they all
accepted, that he was not dying but was simply ill,
and that he only need keep quiet and undergo a
treatment and something very good would result.
He, however, knew that do what they would nothing would come of it, only still more agonizing suffering and death. This deception tortured him—
their not wanting to admit what they all knew and
what he knew, of wanting to lie to him concerning
his terrible condition, and wishing and forcing him
to participate in that lie. Those lies—lies enacted
over him on the eve of his death and destined to
degrade this awful, solemn act to the level of their
visitings, their curtains, their sturgeon for dinner—
were a terrible agony for Ivan Ilych.

The stages of death and dying have been viewed from both a philosophical and a biobehavioral perspective, including symptom management of cachexia and pain, (Kübler-Ross, 1969; Kastenbaum, 1979; Feifel, 1977). Curiously, despite the rank order of causes of death—with cardiovascular disease leading the list—most of the literature concerned with death and dying focuses on death from cancer. Perhaps this is so because, as Sontag (1978) points out, cancer today (as tuberculosis was a century ago) is an inherently mysterious and fearful disease. Because cancers are not readily controllable, excessive psychological meaning becomes attached to the specter of malignancy. We will not attempt to address the many issues related to death and dying. Rather, we will focus on the issue of treatment "noncompliance" in the terminally ill, or the refusal of treatment in end-stage disease. (For a more thorough review of this literature, see Garfield, 1978; Feifel, 1977; Kastenbaum, 1979; Sobel, 1981.)

The dying patient's right to refuse treatment rests fundamentally on the concept of informed consent and the right to self-determination. Legally, the right to refuse treatment— the right to be "let alone"—has been upheld in the courts. Such refusal of treatment on the part of an adult is valid not only in the light of self-determination but also according to the principle of the right of privacy. Such rights are not absolute, of course, as recent court decisions regarding the treatment of minors have made clear. Courts can and do intervene to protect the life of minors when parents' decisions are seen as jeopardizing the child's right to life. In addition, the state has a right to intervene in order to protect its own interest. For example, if the adult refusing treatment has a minor child at home, the courts have the right to order the continuation of reasonable treatment, so that the minor child will be cared for by the parent as long as possible.

Dying is at one level a social process occurring among individuals—the patient, the family, and members of the health care and legal systems. Even the very definition of death is a socially derived one, resting on individual or collective judgment that a brain has ceased to function in support of "meaningful" (value-laden) human life. This decision-making process regarding cessation of "extraordinary" life-sustaining efforts is often a complex one. (And what is "extraordinary" itself becomes a matter of judgment. For example, continuing to feed a long-comatose patient may become an extraordinary act in itself.) In an early analysis of the decision-making process during dying, Miller (1971) examined the management of ten dying patients from the perspectives of physician, staff, family, and patient. Only in two out of the ten cases was there agreement by all parties on the decision to suspend or terminate support efforts. In nine of the ten cases, the medical staff wanted to continue support services; in seven of the cases, the family wished to terminate care. This matter of congruency and the effects of incongruent decisions between family and caregiver is an increasingly important, yet understudied, area.

In the following case, the patient and his family ultimately decided to discontinue active treatment for his clearly terminal condition:

Mr. R., a sixty-two-year-old machinist, was hospitalized for metastatic cancer. For many years he had suffered from disabling rheumatoid arthritis, requiring bilateral hip replacements. Two years before admission, he had had a carcinoma of the colon resected. Since the resected nodes contained tumor, he had also received adjuvant chemotherapy, which he discontinued after a year because of severe vomiting. He felt well until a month before admission, when he developed abdominal and lower back pain, weight loss, and weakness. Evaluation at another hospital was inconclusive. When he developed progressive vomiting and urinary retention, he came to the emergency room. Examination revealed a hard pelvic mass. The patient had mild anemia . . . and slightly elevated liver function tests. A plain film of the abdomen suggested colonic obstruction. An abdominal ultrasound showed a solid pelvic mass and bilateral hydronephrosis. Although there was no tissue confirmation, recurrent metastatic carcinoma was diagnosed. Treatment with narcotics and a nasal gastric tube relieved his discomfort. Urethral catheters allowed a diuresis, but the catheters fell out after two days. An oncology consultant recommended that neither chemotherapy nor radiation was likely to benefit him.

Knowing the impossibility of treating his cancer, the patient and his family refused laboratory tests, antibiotics, transfusions, palliative surgery, and dialysis. They agreed to the use of pain medicine (morphine and an antiemetic parenterally around the clock), nasogastric suction, and intravenous fluids. His mind was clear, and he spoke openly and affectionately with his family about his approaching death [Lo and Jonsen, 1980, p. 107].

Lo and Jonsen, in their discussion of this case, make a distinction between passive euthanasia (withholding further treatments, at the voluntary request of the patient and family, and allowing the patient to die) and active euthanasia (causing to die, or hastening death, in a deliberate fashion). Active euthanasia is currently illegal in the United States. However, the issues are complex. If the distinction is made on the basis of *intent*, advocates of active euthanasia point out that intent is just as present in cases of passive euthanasia. That is, withholding antibiotics for rampant infections also involves intent to let die, to hasten the process of dying, and the active, physical writing out of orders to carry out the intent. On the other hand, those opposed to active euthanasia point out that, once this practice is condoned, it will be very difficult to develop safeguards to limit the policy. The opportunity for mischief and abuse, with resulting widespread social ramifications, would be ultimately uncontrollable: "Would we . . . approve of active [euthanasia] in the next case if the consent were not quite as clear, or if the diagnosis were a little less certain? . . . A wider practice may . . . result from the lowering of psychological or social barriers to killing. Physicians may become less vigilant or careful in their deliberations once their initial resistance has been broken. The cumlative or long-term effects of widespread euthanasia could be a loss of respect for life and a loss of trust by patients for health professionals'' (Lo and Jonsen, 1980, p. 108).

Although the practice of active euthanasia has its advocates, most bioethicists agree with the courts that the opportunities for abuse outweigh any advantage for the deliberate hastening of death that is inevitable in any case. Letting die—and maintaining the patient in comfort and freedom from pain—appears to be the more humane course. But there is little disagreement among the experts that patients at this stage of their illness, including pediatric patients who are faced with either experimental (phase II) treatments or merely supportive care (Nitschke and others, 1982), have the absolute right to withdraw from treatment, even if such withdrawal hastens death. Of course, all patients have this right of self-determination and privacy—the right to be let alone. But in the case of proven therapy for early-stage disease, the medical care establishment may have more obligation to encourage, enhance, and support patient cooperation and compliance with such treatements. In the case of terminal care and phase II trials, the weight of the decision process tips in favor of patient judgment and personal choice reflecting patient and family quality-of-life values.

Behavioral Implications Related to Noncompliance with Cancer Treatments. Since noncompliance with proven treatment in at least early-stage cancer patients contributes indirectly to less than optimal outcome, health care providers should acquaint themselves with techniques for enhancing compliance found in the current literature, even though few studies focusing specifically on cancer patients appear as part of this literature.

Several good reviews of compliance-enhancing technology exist (Becker and Maiman, 1980; Cummings, Becker, Kirscht, and Levin, 1981; Epstein and Cluss, 1982; Haynes, Taylor, and Sackett, 1979). The Becker and Maiman article specifically is a practical guide for utilizing techniques that have proven most effective in assisting patients to comply with treatments. In addition to *altering characteristics of the regimen* where possible (for example, decreasing complexity, duration, costs, and inconvenience and minimizing requirements for massive life-style change), they discuss the use of *patient-provider contracts* as a useful compliance-enhancing technique. Contracts are presumed to enhance compliance by (1) clarifying the relative responsibilities of the parties involved (patients and perhaps their families as well as providers of care) in achieving explicit, agreed-upon goals, and (2) transferring power from provider to patient, which, in turn, affects health-related expectancies (Lewis and Michnich, 1977). Across a wide variety of patient populations, the use of contracts, with built-in rewards for patient success in achieving short-term and long-term goals, and with explicit review and renewal options as part of the contract negotiations, has proved to be a powerful device in optimizing patient cooperation. As Cassileth (1982) concluded in her discussion of active non-compliance and the use of unorthodox therapies, patients who are explicitly involved in the treatment planning may be less likely to turn to alternative treatments.

Social support, particularly support provided by the patient's family, may also influence patient compliance (Dunbar and Stunkard, 1979). When family members can provide rewards for compliant behavior in a contingent, systematic manner, then the efficacy of social support and the efficacy of contingency contracting may, in fact, act in a synergistic rather than an additive fashion.

A Cautionary End Note

Compliance issues are complex—not only across patient populations but within patient populations and across stages of disease, from prevention of illness to terminal care. Little is known specifically about cancer patients' (or physicians') motives to comply or to seek out alternative arrangements to accepted practice. We have begun to map out parameters within patient, physician, and treatment settings that affect the care delivery process aimed at cancer control. We have only begun to understand such behaviors as indirect contributors to cancer outcome.

Steven J. Schleifer
Steven E. Keller
Marvin Stein

5

ϾϾϾϾϾϾϾϾϾϾϾϾ

Central Nervous System Mechanisms and Immunity: Implications for Tumor Response

Both animal and human studies have suggested that psychosocial factors contribute to the development and course of cancer. These factors—including exposure to a variety of stressors, altered mood states, early life experiences, and personality traits—are reviewed elsewhere in this volume, especially in Chapters Three, Six, and Seven.

The evidence suggesting a causal link between psychosocial factors and the development and course of neoplasia has led to much speculation concerning the nature of the biological processes that may be involved. Immune function is one of many factors that might mediate between psychosocial influences and

Note: The authors are members of the staff of the Department of Psychiatry, Mt. Sinai School of Medicine of the City University of New York. Steven J. Schleifer, M.D., is assistant professor of psychiatry; Steven E. Keller, Ph.D., is research associate professor of psychiatry; Marvin Stein, M.D., is Esther and Joseph Klingenstein Professor and chairman of the department.

cancer susceptibility and outcome. This chapter will review evidence suggesting that the brain plays a role in the regulation of immunity and that many of the psychosocial processes associated with cancer growth also influence the immune system. While studies concurrently investigating psychosocial effects on the immune system and on tumor growth are lacking, the accumulated evidence is consistent with a mediating role for altered immunity in the association between psychological and neoplastic processes. Furthermore, immune modulation by the central nervous system (CNS) may provide a link between psychological state, immune function, and the development of pathological states such as neoplasias. Before describing some of the experimental models utilized to investigate psychosocial and CNS effects on immunity, we will briefly review the major components of the immune system.

Immune responses are involved in maintaining the integrity of the organism in relation to foreign substances such as bacteria, viruses, and neoplasias. Exaggerated immune responses directed at the self can also occur, resulting in a variety of autoimmune disorders. Almost all types of immune responses require the participation of one or several subclasses of lymphocytes, which can be found in peripheral blood, the thymus, regional lymph nodes, and the spleen. The immune system can be divided into processes primarily mediated by T lymphocytes, known as cell-mediated immune functions, and those mediated by B lymphocytes, humoral immune processes. Both T and B lymphocytes derive from cells in the bone marrow, with additional maturation of T cells in early life in the thymus. Other cells, such as monocytes, mast cells, and neutrophils, participate as accessory cells in many immune processes. When antigens, which are substances recognized as foreign, attach to specific lymphocytes, lymphocyte proliferation occurs, resulting ultimately in a specific immune response directed at clearing the antigen. Following the primary exposure to an antigen, a subset of memory lymphocytes become programmed to recognize that antigen upon reexposure at a later time. This secondary immune response is more rapid and extensive than the primary response.

The effector function of B cells is mediated by the production of circulating antibodies, which are immunoglobulins
with specificity for a particular antigen. There are five classes
of immunoglobulins in man: IgM, IgG, IgA, IgD, and IgE.
A given antigen may induce the development of one or several
of these classes of antibodies, which tend to be localized to different tissues and have differing functional properties. Humoral
immunity is primarily involved with protection against bacterial
infections. In contrast to B Cells, which secrete circulating immunoglobulins, the T cell participates in immune reactions. T-
cell effects involve cell-to-cell interactions, including cytotoxic
effects on antigen-bearing cells and regulatory effects on the activity of other T and B cells and of other cells involved in immune and inflammatory processes. Cell-mediated immune responses include protection against viral, fungal, and intracellular
bacterial infections and immune surveillance against neoplasia.

Psychosocial Factors and Immunity

Evidence has been accumulating to suggest that stress and
other psychosocial factors associated with cancer risk can also
influence immunity. Of particular importance is the evidence
linking behavioral processes and cell-mediated immunity, which
plays an important role in cancer immunology. However, the
early theories suggesting a major role for the immune system
in protecting against the large majority of cancers have not been
supported by more recent research. It is now believed that the
development and course of only some tumors are restricted by
immune activity and that immune factors may actually stimulate
tumor growth under certain conditions (Fox, 1978). This diver-
sity of effects is not surprising considering current concepts of
immunity as a network of interacting systems subject to inadequate or exaggerated responses to antigenic challenge. It is now
believed that the balance between the activity of helper and suppressor regulatory T cells is critical to the maintenance of effective immunity. To date, most studies of the brain and behavior in relation to the immune system have utilized very
general measures of immune activity and have not investigated

the effects of CNS processes on many of the specific components of the immune response. Conclusions to be derived from these studies in relation to the role of brain, behavior, and immunity in clinically significant pathological processes such as tumor growth must therefore be considered tentative at present.

Stress and Humoral Immune Responses

A variety of stressors have been found to alter humoral immune responses in animals, usually suppressing the response. Studies utilizing a variety of species (Petrovski, 1961; Hill, Greer, and Felsenfeld, 1967; Vessey, 1964) have found that the production of specific antibody is suppressed by stressful environmental stimuli, such as noise, light, movement, or housing conditions. However, other stressors, such as repeated low-voltage electric shock, seem to enhance antibody responses (Solomon, 1969; Hirata-Hibi, 1967). More recent studies have tended to support the observation that, while acute exposure to a stressor can suppress humoral immune responses, repeated exposure results in an apparent adaptation of the animals to the stressor and, in some cases, an enhanced response (Monjan and Collector, 1977). The complexity of stress effects on humoral immunity has been demonstrated in studies that found differential effects of different stresses on antibody responses in rats, depending on the sex of the animal (Joasoo and McKenzie, 1976). Only a few reports suggest that there may be alterations in humoral immunity in relation to psychological conditions in man (Fessel, 1962; Pettingale, Greer, and Tee, 1977), and further research in this area is required.

Several studies have found that exposure to stressful life experiences can alter the functional capacity of T lymphocytes to respond to mitogens, which are substances capable of nonspecifically inducing lymphocyte proliferation without prior antigen sensitization. In man, brief effects on T-cell mitogen responses lasting no more than several days have been found following sleep deprivation (Palmblad and others, 1979), running a marathon (Eskola and others, 1978), or space flight (Kimzey, Johnson, Ritzman, and Mengel, 1976). The death of a spouse, among the most stressful of commonly occurring life events (Holmes and Masuda, 1974), has been associated with a more prolonged suppression of T-lymphocyte function. In 1977 Bartrop and co-workers in Australia described decreased lymphocyte stimulation responses to mitogens in a group of bereaved spouses seven to ten weeks after bereavement. We have studied the husbands of women who ultimately died of breast cancer and found that lymphocyte responses to mitogens were significantly suppressed in these men during the first two months following the death of the spouse, compared with prebereavement levels (Schleifer and others, 1983). Follow-up of the subjects during the remainder of the postbereavement year demonstrated a return of lymphocyte activity to prebereavement levels for most but not all of the husbands.

There is also evidence that clinical depression is associated with altered lymphocyte function. Kronfol, Silva, and Greden (1983) found that melancholic patients had lower lymphcyte responses to the mitogens PHA, ConA, and PWM than groups of nonmelancholic psychiatric patients and normal controls. We have conducted a series of studies to determine whether depressive disorders are associated with altered immunity (Schleifer and others, 1984). Mitogen-induced lymphocyte stimulation responses and the number of peripheral blood lymphocytes were measured in a groups of medication-free inpatients with major depressive disorder. Lymphocyte stimulation responses to PHA, ConA, and PWM were significantly lower in the hospitalized depressives than in age- and sex-matched controls. The total number of lymphocytes was significantly lower in the depressed subjects than in the controls, as was the absolute number of both T and B cells. These findings demonstrate that the functional activity of the lymphocyte, as well as the number of circulating immunocompetent cells, is decreased in individuals hospitalized with major depressive disorder.

It remains to be determined whether the immune changes found in the bereaved and in depressed patients are causally related to the increased morbidity and mortality reported in those groups. Several studies have suggested that loss often precedes the onset of lymphoid and other cancers (LeShan, 1959; Greene,

1966) and that states of depression predispose to cancer onset (Shekelle and others, 1981; Hagnell, 1966). Since conjugal bereavement regularly elicits depressive mood states (Clayton, 1979), it may be that immune changes following losses such as bereavement or in persons experiencing depression are associated with an increased risk for neoplasia. Causal relationships between these factors, however, remain to be demonstrated.

Several studies have recently demonstrated that the psychological state of an animal can influence cancer growth. In these studies groups of animals were exposed to the same total amount of electric shock, but only one group of animals was able to terminate the stressor—both for itself and for a second, yoked, group. Under these conditions mice or rats who received the shock in an unpredictable and uncontrollable manner showed increased tumor growth compared with nonshock controls, but animals who were able to control the shock had no increment in tumor growth (Sklar and Anisman, 1979; Visintainer, Volpicelli, and Seligman, 1982). Using a similar behavioral paradigm, Laudenslager and colleagues (1983) found that rats who were unable to control the presentation of a shock had suppressed lymphocyte responses following exposure to the stressor, although animals who received the same total amount of shock but were able to terminate the stressor had no suppression of mitogen response. These observations suggest that the ability to cope with a stressor can mitigate the negative impact of that experience, both on immunity and on tumor growth.

Early life experiences, which can modify susceptibility to tumor growth in animals (Ader and Friedman, 1965; Levine and Cohen, 1959), have also been found to influence immune function. For example, Keller and his associates (1983a), studying the effects on T-cell function of premature maternal separation in rats, found a decrease in the number of peripheral blood lymphocytes and in mitogen responses in the adult animals that had been prematurely weaned. Moreover, increased spontaneously occurring respiratory infections were found later in life in the prematurely weaned animals. Other researchers (Michaut and others, 1981) have found that premature weaning can suppress humoral immune responses in mice.

In summary, many of the psychosocial factors that have been related to cancer susceptibility can also influence T-cell function. To delineate the nature of these interrelationships, further studies with more comprehensive immune assessments and concomitant measures of both immunity and tumor growth are required. An important related question concerns the role of the brain in modulating immune processes. The demonstration of neuroimmunomodulation has provided support for the notion that psychosocial processes may modulate immunity directly, as a result of altered brain states, and not merely indirectly, through changes in diet, activity, or sleep.

Brain Effects on Immunity

While early immunologists considered the possibility that the central nervous system (CNS) might be involved in immune processes, this area of investigation subsequently received little attention until the past several decades. Systematic investigation of the relationship between the brain and immune function was initiated in a series of studies concerned with the effects of brain lesions on lethal anaphylaxis. Anaphylaxis is a humoral immune response related to severe allergic and asthmatic reactions in man. In experimental models of anaphylaxis, an animal is sensitized to an antigen that includes a specific antibody (usually IgE or IgG), which attaches to cells such as mast cells in the lung. When the animal is reexposed to the antigen, an immune reaction between the antigen and the tissue-fixed antibody ensues. This reaction results in the release of a variety of chemical agents from the mast cells; these agents induce bronchiolar constriction and the secretion of fluids, which can result in wheezing, respiratory distress, and asphyxiation.

In 1958 Freedman and Fenichel reported that bilateral midbrain lesions inhibited anaphylactic shock in the guinea pig; and Filipp and Szentivanyi demonstrated that lethal anaphylactic shock in the guinea pig and in the rabbit can be prevented by bilateral focal lesions in the hypothalamus. The hypothalamus— because of its critical role in the regulation of a wide range of peripheral functions, including endocrine, neurotransmitter, and visceral processes, and behavior—is an area of the brain of particular interest for the study of CNS and immune relationships. Endocrine and neurotransmitter activity has been shown to participate in the modulation of immune processes.

We have investigated brain effects on immunity, utilizing an experimental model in which bilateral electrolytic lesions are placed in the anterior, median, or posterior basal hypothalamus of either rats or guinea pigs. The animals were sensitized with antigen one week following the operative procedure and then reexposed to the antigen to induce anaphylaxis four weeks later. In our initial studies, we found that anterior but not posterior hypothalamic lesions inhibited development of lethal anaphylaxis in the rat (Luparello, Stein, and Park, 1964). Significant protection against lethal anaphylaxis induced by a variety of sensitizing antigens was also found in guinea pigs with electrolytic lesions in the anterior hypothalamus (Macris, Schiavi, Camerino, and Stein, 1970; Schiavi, Macris, Camerino, and Stein, 1975). Median and posterior hypothalamic lesions had no significant protective effect (Macris, Schiavi, Camerino, and Stein, 1970). While these studies indicated that antigen-induced anaphylaxis may be modified by hypothalamic lesions, the mechanisms involved in these effects require clarification. Protection against anaphylaxis may have been related to altered antibody production, to nonimmune changes in the production of chemical mediators of anaphylaxis in the lung, to altered target organ responsivity, or to a combination of effects.

A number of investigators have attempted to demonstrate changes in the levels of circulating antibodies following brain lesions, but findings from these studies have been inconsistent. Some studies found decreased antibody production in animals with hypothalamic lesions (Korneva and Khai, 1964; Filipp and Szentivanyi, 1958; Macris, Schiavi, Camerino, and Stein, 1970; Tyrey and Nalbandov, 1972), while others found no change in antibody levels following placement of hypothalamic lesions (Ado and Goldstein, 1973; Thrasher, Bernardis, and Cohen, 1971; Schiavi, Macris, Camerino, and Stein, 1975). These differing findings may have resulted from technical differences among the antibody assays, resulting in differing levels of sensitivity to immune effects. However, hypothalamic lesions may affect only some types of humoral immune responses and only under certain conditions of sensitization and challenge. Antibody studies have utilized different animal species, a wide range of sensitizing and test doses, variable time schedules, and different antigens; and, in some cases, different types of immune responses may be involved. For example, hypothalamic effects on antibody production by B cells have been more readily demonstrated with antigens that require the participation of T-helper cells in the response. Perhaps B cells are not directly sensitive to brain and behavioral effects, and perhaps the effects of hypothalamic lesions on lethal anaphylaxis are due to nonimmune aspects of anaphylaxis. Several studies found that hypothalamic lesions alter the release of chemical mediators of anaphylaxis, such as histamine and prostaglandins, as well as target organ responses to these agents (Mathe, Yen, Sohn, and Kemper, 1978; Whittier and Orr, 1962; Szentivanyi and Szekely, 1958; Schiavi, Adams, and Stein, 1966). The effects of hypothalamic lesions on anaphylaxis may also be related to changes in vagal parasympathetic activity (Gold, 1973; Koller, 1968; Mills and Widdicombe, 1970; Parker, 1973).

We have recently completed a study which indicates that changes in specific immune functions play an important role in the protective effect of anterior hypothalamic lesions on anaphylaxis. In this study guinea pigs were sensitized to an antigen prior to, rather than following, placement of anterior hypothalamic lesions. No differences were found between lesioned and control animals in the incidence of lethal anaphylaxis, suggesting that the protective effect of anterior hypothalamic lesions found in our previous studies resulted from altered antigen sensitization. Studies by Besedovsky and co-workers have provided further evidence of a specific relationship between the hypothalamus and a humoral immune response. They found an increase in the firing rate of neurons in the ventromedial nuclei of the hypothalamus in rats (Besedovsky and Sorkin, 1977), as well as altered hypothalamic noradrenergic activity (Besedovsky and others, 1983) at the peak of an immune response. These results demonstrate the presence of a feedback loop between the immune response and the hypothalamus.

Brain effects on cell-mediated immune processes have also been studied. In 1970 we reported that anterior hypothalamic lesions in the guinea pig suppressed skin test responses to tuberculin antigen (Macris, Schiavi, Camerino, and Stein, 1970). Median and posterior hypothalamic lesions did not alter the response. Other workers reported that a lesion involving a large part of the hypothalamus in the rat resulted in a decreased skin test response to other antigens and that hypothalamic stimulation enhanced the responses (Jankovic, Jovanova, and Markovic, 1979). We have also found that hypothalamic lesions in the guinea pig alter lymphcyte activity measured *in vitro* (Keller and others, 1980). As in our studies of humoral immunity, bilateral electrolytic lesions were placed in the anterior hypothalamus one week prior to sensitization with antigen. While no differences were found in the numbers of total lymphocytes, B cells, or T cells among the various groups, the hypothalamic lesions suppressed lymphocyte stimulation by tuberculin antigen (PPD) and by the T-cell mitogen phytohemagglutinin (PHA) when the lymphocytes were cultured in whole blood. These findings established that the hypothalamus can directly influence lymphocyte function. In contrast, the lesioned animals did not differ from controls in tuberculin or mitogen responses when the lymphocytes were isolated and cultured separately from other blood compoents. This finding suggests that the lesions do not impair the primary acquisition of immunity to an antigen but rather modify the secondary expression of cell-mediated immune processes. In addition, the absence of an effect in cultures of lymphocytes isolated from other blood components suggests that the modulating effect of anterior hypothalamic lesions on the T lymphocyte may be related to humoral factors or to changes in accessory cells, such as macrophages, monocytes, erythrocytes, and platelets (Bach and Hirschhorn, 1965; Ferguson, Schmidtke, and Simmons, 1976).

In another experimental model, Roszman and co-workers (Cross, Markesbery, Brooks, and Roszman, 1980) have demonstrated short-term effects of brain lesions on cell-mediated immune function in the rat. Animals with bilateral anterior hypothalamic lesions were compared with controls four to fourteen days after placement of the lesions. Four days following the procedure, both lymphocyte and spleen cell numbers were lower in the animals with hypothalamic lesions; however, by fourteen days the effect was no longer apparent. Similarly, mitogen responses of spleen cell suspensions were suppressed four days after placement of the hypothalamic lesions but not at seven or fourteen days. In contrast, lesions in other areas of the limbic system, the hippocampus and amygdaloid complex, were found to increase mitogen responsivity. The investigators further found that all the short-term effects of brain lesions on immunity could be reversed by hypophysectomy, suggesting a role for endocrine alterations in the effects. It remains to be determined whether the mechanisms involved in these short-term immune effects of hypothalamic lesions, lasting only several days, are similar to those mediating the immune effects found in our studies, which persisted for at least five weeks after placement of hypothalamic lesions. It is also not known whether either or both of these neuroimmunological processes are involved in mediating the effects of stress and other psychosocial factors on immunity.

Further evidence of brain effects on cell-mediated immunity have come from clincial studies. Brooks and co-workers (Brooks, Netsky, Normansell, and Horwitz, 1972) studied patients with benign and malignant primary intracranial tumors who showed no systemic evidence of serious illness or malnutrition. In contrast with healthy controls, patients with brain tumors showed diminished skin test responses to a variety of antigens and lower lymphocyte stimulation responses to antigens and T-cell mitogens. In addition, more than two thirds of the patients could not be sensitized to the chemical antigen DNCB, whereas healthy control subjects were all successfully sensitized to the antigen. These findings indicated a deficit in the patients' ability to mount a specific T-cell response.

Mediation of Brain and Behavioral Effects on Immune Function

Investigation of possible mechanisms of brain and behavioral effects on immune function have focused on the hypothalamus, with particular emphasis on the neuroendocrine axis.

Hypophysectomy can depress both antibody production and skin test responses in rats (Nagy and Berczi, 1978) and, as noted above, can abolish some of the effects of brain lesions on immunity. Studies by Filipp and Mess (1969) further suggested that the protective effect of hypothalamic lesions on anaphylaxis may be related to changes in a number of endocrine functions. They found that thyroxine and an inhibitor of adrenocortical synthesis each partially restored the sensitivity to anaphylaxis of guinea pigs with hypothalamic lesions. Other studies have demonstrated the role of the thyroid in enhancing immune processes in the rat, mouse, and guinea pig (Denckla, 1978; Leger and Masson, 1947; Nilzen, 1955), and thyroid activity has been reported to be altered in depression and following stress in man (Whybrow and Prange, 1981; Loosen and Prange, 1982).

Changes in corticosteroid levels may have a major role in the mediation of the effects of behavioral and brain states on immunity. There is considerable evidence demonstrating modulation of a wide variety of immune parameters by pharmacological and physiological doses of corticosteroids (Claman, 1972; Fauci, 1975; Fauci and Dale, 1975; Thomson, McMahon, and Nugent, 1980). These observations have tended to support the hypothesis that adrenal hormones are primary mediators of psychosocial and CNS effects on the immune system (Riley, 1981). Several studies of stress effects on the immune response have measured adrenocortical activity and immune function in parallel. An early study by Marsh and Rasmussen (1960) found that stress in mice was accompanied by adrenal hypertrophy, lymphopenia, and a slowly developing involution of the thymus and spleen, associated with increased susceptibility to viral infection. Several other groups found increased corticosteroid levels concomitant with suppressed immune function in mice (Gisler, 1974; Monjan and Collector, 1977), although studies of cortisol levels in relation to stress effects on immunity in man have been equivocal (Eskola and others, 1978; Bartrop and others, 1977). One study found that the antibody titer depression following anterior hypothalamic lesions in the rat can be significantly blocked by either hypophysectomy or adrenalectomy (Tyrey and Nalbandov, 1972). While these studies suggest an association between stress, the brain, cortisol, and immunity, cortisol secretion may not be causally related to induced changes in immunity, since the cortisol and immune effects may be independent, unrelated concomitants of stress.

Two recent studies that compared stress effects in intact and adrenalectomized animals have demonstrated that corticosteroids are required for some but not all stress effects on immunity. Blecha, Kelley, and Satterlee (1982) found, in mice, that stress effects on skin test responses to sheep red blood cell antigens, but not to the chemical antigen DNFB, required an intact adrenal. We have found that stress-induced lymphopenia in rats requires intact adrenal function but that suppression of lymphocyte responses to mitogens following stress can be elicited despite the absence of the adrenal (Keller and others, 1983b). It thus appears that there are adrenal-independent as well as adrenal-dependent stress effects on immunity and that stress-induced modulation of immunity is a complex phenomenon involving several, if not multiple, mechanisms.

A variety of other hormonal systems may also play a role in the psychosocial and CNS influences on immunity. Growth hormone (GH) is released in response to various stressors (Brown and Reichlin, 1972), is regulated by anterior hypothalamic functions (Alpert, Brawer, Patel, and Reichlin, 1976; Rice, Abe, and Critchlow, 1978), and can enhance the immune response (Gisler, 1974; Denckla, 1978). Testosterone, which appears to have a suppressive effect on immune function (Wyle and Kent, 1977; Mendelsohn, Multer, and Bernheim, 1977), has been reported to be suppressed by a number of stressful conditions (Mason, 1975; Repcekova and Mikulaj, 1977), while levels may increase in other situations (Mason, 1975). Androgens and estrogens can suppress skin test responses (Kappas, Jones, and Roitt, 1963), while gonadectomy in male and female guinea pigs may enhance cell-mediated immune responses (Kittas and Henry, 1979). Estrogens may increase humoral immune responses to antigens (Eidinger and Garrett, 1972; Thanavala, Rao, and Thakur, 1973).

Influences other than hormonal may be involved in CNS regulation of immunity. As noted, hypothalamic lesions in hypophysectomized rats have been found to induce an increase in the number of thymic lymphocytes and a decrease in mitogen responses (Cross, Markesbery, Brooks, and Roszman, 1980). A direct link between the CNS and immunocompetent tissues has been suggested by the demonstration of nerve endings in the thymus, spleen, and lymph nodes (Calvo, 1968; Bulloch and Moore, 1980; Giron, Crutcher, and Davis, 1980; Williams and others, 1980). Furthermore, adrenergic and cholinergic receptors have been identified on the lymphocyte surface (Bourne, Lichtenstein, and Melmon, 1974; Pochet, Delesperse, Gauseet, and Collet, 1979); and epinephrine and norepinephrine, which increase in response to stressful stimuli (Mason and others, 1961; Frankenhaeuser, 1971), can suppress humoral and cell-mediated immune responses. Stressful life experiences have also been found to induce elevations in free fatty acids, cholesterol, and uric acid. These agents all may have immunosuppressive effects (Criep, 1969; Dilman, 1977). Of particular interest has been recent research demonstrating that a wide range of peptides under neural control appear to be secreted in response to stress. Some of these—such as endorphin and other opioids, somatostatin, and substance P—have been found to alter a variety of immune responses (Weber and Pert, 1984). For example, Shavit and co-workers (1984) recently found a suppression of natural killer cell activity following exposure to foot shock in rats and demonstrated that the stress-induced suppression was mediated by opioid mechanisms.

In conclusion, psychosocial and CNS processes can modify both humoral and cell-mediated immune processes. An extensive network of endocrine and autonomic processes may be involved in these effects. The multiple pathways linking limbic and higher cortical areas with the hypothalamus suggest that the hypothalamus may be of central importance in mediating psychosocial influences on endocrine, neurotransmitter, and immune functions. Further research is required to determine whether interactions among the hypothalamus, the neuroendocrine system, and the immune system, in response to psychosocial factors, alter the development and course of neoplastic disorders.

6

Marc E. Lippman

Psychosocial Factors and the Hormonal Regulation of Tumor Growth

Over the past few years, increasing attention has focused on the possibility that psychological factors influence the rate of human tumor progression. The notion that malignant tumors invariably represent completely unregulated proliferation of neoplastic cells is now known to be vastly oversimplified. An extraordinary expansion of our knowledge of the ways in which many human tumors can be influenced by their environment has provided a very attractive set of mechanisms for understanding how a variety of humoral, endocrine, immune, and psychological factors can profoundly alter tumor growth rates. The information presented in this chapter may permit a rational classification of ways in which such psychological factors potentially alter tumor growth. In addition, the concepts of tumor cell biology that will be discussed should permit a closer linkage of observed rates of tumor progession with psychological factors.

Much of this information is summarized in the model shown in Figure 3. This model presents various environmental

Note: Marc E. Lippman, M.D., is head of the breast cancer section, Medicine Branch, National Cancer Institute, Bethesda, Md.

Figure 3. Interaction of Psychic and Endocrine Factors with Progression of Neoplastic Disease.

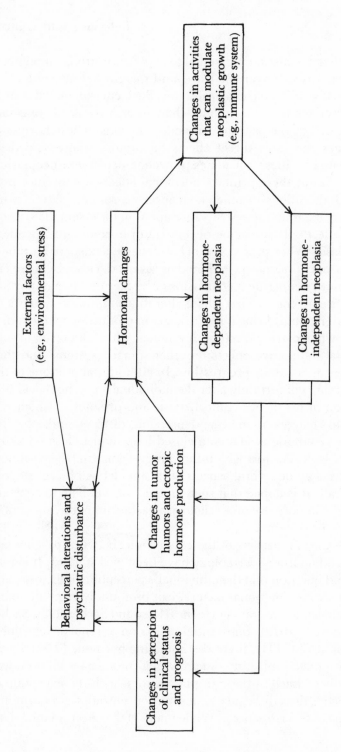

Source: Reprinted by permission of the publisher from S. Levy (ed.), *Biological Mediators of Behavior and Disease: Neoplasia*, p. 56, copyright 1982 by Elsevier Science Publishing Co., Inc.

stimuli that cause an individual to experience strong emotions—such as stress, anger, or fear—and thereby influence that individual's basic psychological status. Such environmental stimuli can produce many hormonal changes as a result of transduction through the psychoneuroendocrine axis. These hormonal changes can have direct effects on tumors whose growth is regulated by these hormones (hormone-dependent neoplasia). In addition, these primary hormonal effects may induce profound alterations in other noncancerous somatic systems, including the immune system. Alterations in these somatic systems may affect both hormone-dependent or hormone-independent neoplasia. When progression of hormone-dependent or hormone-independent neoplasia is altered or reversed, either by these endogenous endocrine mechanisms or by therapy, two important results may ensue. First, these alterations in tumor viability or growth rate may bring about changes in production by the tumor of growth factors and ectopic hormones, which can result in substantial interactive effects on other somatic systems and thus further alter tumor progression. In addition, alterations in the neoplasm will certainly alter the individual's psychological perception of his or her clinical status and prognosis, which will lead to changes in anxiety, depression, distress, and other responsive emotions. Thus, a closed-loop model closely linking psychological factors with tumor progression can be envisioned. In this chapter several aspects of this model will be considered in detail. It is hoped that such an analysis will help to substantiate the importance of psychological factors in modifying human tumor progression.

Certain aspects of the connections between psychic factors and neuroendocrinology have been well studied. It is now beyond question that the individual's perception of distress, and other strong emotional factors, can profoundly regulate many hypothalamic-pituitary hormones (Rose and Sacher, 1981; Sacher and Baron, 1979). Substantial effects on adrenocorticotrophic hormone (ACTH), thyroid-stimulating hormone (TSH), gonadotrophins, prolactin, and growth hormone have all been well described. Each of these trophic factors, with the exception of prolactin, directly regulates plasma concentrations of hormones that have diverse actions. While many of the effects of these hormones are metabolic, sex and adrenal steroids as well as thyroid hormone have major effects on behavior (Miller and Spratt, 1979). In addition, all these hormones that are under neuroendocrine control (estrogens, androgens, progestins, glucocorticoids, insulin-like growth factor, prolactin, and iodothyronines) either directly regulate neoplastic cell growth or alter concentrations or activities of other hormones that affect cancer cells (Lippman, Strobl, and Allegra, 1980). The picture is even more complicated than this, however. First, a great many brain peptides, which are either less well characterized or of unknown function, are also secreted into the general circulation. These include the melanocyte-stimulating hormones and the enkephalins. In addition, *in vivo*, it is impossible to alter the level of a single hormone without having profound effects on the activities and concentrations of many others. For example, administration of estrogens is associated with substantial effects on gonadotrophins, prolactin, growth hormone, and thyroid hormones. Some of these effects appear to be direct (for example, sex steroid suppression of follicle-stimulating hormone, or FSH), while others may occur through such diverse mechanisms as alterations in hormone metabolism or hormone-binding moieties (Kakidani and others, 1982).

A host of recently described tumor growth factors may also be altered by changes in estrogen concentration (Ikeda and Sirbasku, 1984). Many tumors are clearly capable of secreting their own exogenous growth factors, which may function as either autocrine or paracrine regulators of cell function. Autocrine regulators are secreted substances that influence the growth of the secreting cells themselves, whereas paracrine factors influence the growth or properties of cells around the secreting cells. For example, all neoplastic cells are capable of secreting paracrine growth factors, such as angiogenesis factors, which are able to induce the proliferation of normal endothelial cells surrounding the tumor. Were it not for this growth factor production, there would be no clinical evidence of malignancy because the tumor cells would be unable to meet their nutritional needs. A particularly interesting example is provided by occasional positive responses to endocrine therapy seen in human breast cancers that apparently lack hormone receptors to mediate endocrine responses. While there are many potential explanations for this phenomenon, one possibility is based on the observation that most breast cancers are heterogeneous with respect to many biochemical properties. A few hormone-dependent cells (insufficient to score positive in a hormone receptor assay) may, through their secretion of paracrine factors, alter the behavior of the entire tumor when an endocrine treatment is applied. It is now clear that frequently the regulation of secretion of such locally acting growth factors is under the control of systemic endocrine function, which, as just mentioned, is in turn influenced by emotions and perceptions. Thus, there can be no question whatsoever that psychological factors can profoundly alter the endocrine milieu.

Effects of Hormone-Dependent Neoplasia

For nearly a century, it has been recognized that some tumors are hormone dependent. For most of this time, attention has classically focused on tumors of the endometrium, prostate, and breast and or leukemia and lymphoma. We, too, will begin our discussion with these, but, as will emerge shortly, this is clearly an inappropriately limited description of the extent of human tumors that should be considered hormone dependent.

Female endometrium is the classic example of a hormone-dependent tissue. Throughout normal menstrual life, it undergoes cyclical changes under the direct control of ovarian estrogen and progesterone secretion. In the absence of estrogenic stimulation, uterine cancer is essentially unknown. Progestins are capable of profound antimitotic effects on normal endometrium, and in approximately one third of cases progestins are capable of inducing regressions of established endometrial cancer. Response is well correlated with the presence of specific progestin receptors in tumor biopsies. Thus, epidemiological, pathophysiological, and clinical data all verify the hormone-dependent nature of at least some endometrial cancers.

The data for breast cancer are equally convincing. In the nineteenth century, Beatson (1896) described the regression of breast cancer in several patients following the removal of their ovaries. The only well-documented "spontaneous" regressions of breast cancer have apparently been associated with metastatic involvement of the ovaries by breast cancer, leading to their eventual destruction and thereby the removal of the significant source of estrogens. Epidemiological data suggesting hormonal factors in the etiology of breast cancer are overwhelmingly convincing (Kelsey and others, 1978). The female-to-male ratio of the disease is 100 to 1. Women with primary ovarian failure without estrogen replacement have an incidence of breast cancer approximating that of men. Other evidence includes the critical links of increased breast cancer risk to early menarche, late age at first full-term pregnancy, late menopause, and increased height and weight. As with endometrial cancer, approximately one third of women with established breast cancer will have beneficial responses when endocrine therapies are given (Lippman, 1981). In the context of the preceding comments, one would assume that removal of estrogens (in the form of castration or adrenalectomy) or the administration of antiestrogens would be effective treatments; however, for reasons that are incompletely understood, progestins, androgens, massive doses of estrogens, and possibly antiprolactin drugs are also useful therapy in some patients. Multiple responses to sequential endocrine therapies are not uncommon.

Recent work from several laboratories has shown that some human breast cancers have receptors for or responses to not only estrogens but also androgens, glucocorticoids, progestins, prolactin, insulin, insulin-like growth factor 1, epidermal growth factor, iodothyronines, retinoids, calcitonin, and vitamin D^3. How these numerous hormones may alter growth *in vivo* and how they may interact with one another is at present almost completely unexplored. This ever increasing array of hormones and growth factors that influence either growth or phenotypical expression in breast cancer (as well as numerous other neoplasms) increases the number of ways in which neuroendocrine changes, in part induced by external stimuli, can alter cancer progression.

The human prostate is also a well-known hormone-responsive organ (Huggins and Hodges, 1941). In the absence

of puberty, prostate cancer never develops. While it was originally thought that perhaps only two thirds of prostate cancers
were responsive to androgens for their growth, recent studies
with total endocrine ablation therapies, using antiandrogens
combined with LHRH analogs, have suggested that nearly 100
percent of patients may initially have hormone-dependent tumors. Once again, a rich body of evidence suggests that hormone responsivity of prostate is not restricted simply to androgens; important direct effects of estrogens and prolactin should
be considered as well (Lippman, 1985). Our knowledge of other
potential prostatic growth factors and their central modulation
by behavioral cues is very limited.

Finally, in the classic grouping of hormone-dependent
neoplasia, one must include the hematological malignancies.
Glucocorticoids have long been known to have profound effects
on the progression of varying proportions of patients with leukemia and lymphoma, largely depending on specific diagnosis
(Borthwick and Bell, 1978). For example, childhood acute lymphoblastic leukemia is almost invariably responsive to glucocorticoids, and they remain a critical component in the multidrug
chemotherapy regimens that have been successful in treating
this disease. Many other hematological malignancies are hormonally responsive to a varying extent. Responsivity has been
correlated with the presence of specific glucocorticoid receptor
sites. Spontaneous regressions of leukemia have been reported
in association with major emotional upheavals. It is worth noting
that concentrations of glucocorticoids sufficient to saturate specific leukemic blood cell receptors, and thereby induce inhibition of division or cell death, are only minimally above circulating concentrations and are certainly achievable as part of the
stress response in some individuals (Lippman, Yarbro, and
Leventhal, 1978). A striking and very moving example is provided by the composer Béla Bartók. While he lay dying from
leukemia, he was approached by Serge Koussevitsky, conduc-
tor of the Boston Symphony Orchestra, who offered him a com-
mission for an orchestral work. Bartók went into a spontaneous
remission over the next few weeks, and the remission persisted
until the work was complete.

Glucocorticoids of course exert profound regulatory effects on the entire normal immune system as well as on some neoplastic cells derived from this system. Given the equally well-known interaction between stress and plasma glucocorticoid concentrations, it requires no great leap to imagine exogenously derived psychic perturbations as influencing the progression of this class of diseases.

Over the past decade, extraordinary success has been achieved in defining growth conditions required for proliferation of many neoplastic cells in culture. For many years it was traditional to supplement medium containing essential amino acids and nutrients with various concentrations of fetal calf serum. The exact role of such serum supplementation was unclear. Largely through the pioneering works of Sato and his colleagues, it has been learned that serum supplementation is critically important as a source of specific hormones and growth factors (Sato, 1980). Using painstaking means, Sato and associates have been able to define the exact growth requirements for numerous cell lines in culture. What emerges is that specific "cocktails" of hormones and growth factors will permit the growth of almost all cell lines thus far studied in culture without a need for additional serum supplementation. The relevance of this observation for the present discussion lies in the fact that virtually all cell lines thus turn out to be "hormone dependent." For example, Carney and colleagues (1981) have shown that small-cell carcinoma of the lung (not traditionally considered a hormone-dependent tumor) can readily be cultivated in defined medium containing hydrocortisone, insulin, transferrin, estradiol, and selenium. And Moody and colleagues (1981) have shown that many small-cell carcinoma cell lines secrete bombesin (a peptide initially found in frog skin). Some small-cell carcinoma cells (but not necessarily those that manufacture and secrete bombesin) require bombesin for proliferation. In very exciting preliminary experiments, Moody and his colleagues found that monoclonal antibody directed against bombesin was able to block the growth of small-cell carcinoma cells both *in vitro* and *in vivo* in nude mice. In a similar way, a large number of cell types can now be grown in completely defined medium in which suitable (and frequently very complicated) hormonal and growth factor supplementation has been provided. Such studies support conclusively that these tumors are responsive to hormones for their growth.

However, the fact that an exogeneously added hormone is able to stimulate the growth of these cells in no way suggests that the specific hormone used *in vitro* is the hormone operative *in vivo*. Many hormones are capable of cross-reacting with other receptors. For example, some transforming growth factors cross-react perfectly with epidermal growth factor receptor. A host of insulin-like growth factors can often cross-react with the insulin receptor, and vice versa; high concentrations of androgen can bind to the estrogen receptor; and many progestins can bind to both glucocorticoid and androgen receptor. Furthermore, different hormones acting through entirely different receptors may stimulate the same pathway. Thus, high concentrations of insulin added to the medium may be required for growth but may not be the specific growth factor responsible *in vivo*. Clearly, such studies are in their infancy but suggest that probably all tumors depend to some extent on specific hormonal factors or growth factors in their environment for their continued proliferation.

By considering only the effects of hormones on growth, one misses many other important effects of hormones on tumors. Many of these effects may dramatically (though indirectly) affect the progression of disease. If either differentiation or altered expression of cell surface antigens is induced, interaction of tumor with surrounding stroma and host effector cells may be greatly modified. Such cell surface antigenic effects can influence immune recognition, invasion potential, and metastatic seeding, to mention but a few possibilities. The difficulty with most currently available animal and cell culture model systems is that they primarily monitor growth of a primary tumor mass or crude survival without assessing more subtle aspects of tumor progression.

Thus far, we have considered the impact of hormone changes on tumors directly. We have emphasized the fact that not only are the classically hormone-dependent tumors potential targets for hormonal alterations, but in fact the biology of most tumors is likely to be directly altered by hormonal effects.

Hormonal Effects on Other Somatic Systems

Progression of human neoplasia represents far more than a continued exponential growth of an isolated malignant cell population. Tumors are also made up of varying amounts of normal stroma, or supporting tissue. All the vasculature in a tumor represents tumor-induced proliferation of normal and epithelial cells. Tumors are frequently infiltrated with leukocytes and a variety of immunocompetent cells. Tumors are made up of varying proportions of cells that are being shed in either a viable or a nonviable state. In the nonviable state, cells may be potentially clonogenic or of limited continued replicative potential. Growth potential or lack of it may be determined as much by changes induced in the host as by any direct effects on the neoplasm itself. It has long been known that variations in glucocorticoid concentrations in the physiological range may have substantial impact on gross evidence of immune functioning. In addition, glucocorticoids alter cell adhesiveness and metastatic potential. Cortisone in combination with heparin profoundly depresses tumor-induced angiogenesis, and subsequent lack of blood vessel growth results in tumor regression (Folkman and Haudenschild, 1980). Hormonal changes can also affect the synthetic potential and functioning of many other organs. For example, estrogens induce increases in thyroid-binding globulin, which is synthesized in the liver. Under certain circumstances this increase may induce a decrease in biologically available thyroid hormone.

The importance of these effects on nontarget tissues cannot be overemphasized. For example, it has long been known that estrogen-recepter-positive tumors respond to antiestrogen therapy (McGuire, 1980). However, up to 10 percent of apparently estrogen-receptor-negative tumors also respond to antiestrogen therapy. Some of these apparently paradoxical responses are undoubtedly due to tumor heterogeneity and laboratory error. But even if the tumor is not a direct target of antiestrogen action, normal tissues—such as liver and pituitary—are; thus, antiestrogen treatment can alter many other hormone and growth factor concentrations to which the tumor may be sensitive.

These hormonal effects on other normally functioning somatic systems may obviously alter the rate of progression not only of classically hormone-dependent neoplasms but of virtually any other neoplasm as well. A single example may help to illustrate this point. For many years it was known that androgen administered to male rodents would cause mammary gland regression. However, it took the ingenious experiments of Kratochwil and colleagues (Durnberger and others, 1978) to show that this regression is the result of androgen induction of a mammary gland regression factor produced by surrounding fibroblasts. The investigators transplanted either normal breast buds or breast buds derived from mice with testicular ferminiza-tion (tfm) into normal mice or other mice with tfm. Normal breasts or breasts from tfm mice regressed when transplanted into normal hosts. Normal and tfm breasts were unresponsive to androgens when transplanted into stroma on tfm mice. Thus, by interposing the response of a nonmalignant but hormonally responsive tissue, one may imagine how hormonal changes in-duced by environmental stimuli may influence not only hor-mone-dependent neoplasia but so-called hormone-independent neoplasia as well.

Consequences of Hormone-Induced Changes in Neoplasia

As previously mentioned, hormones may evoke profound changes not only in hormone-dependent neoplasms but also in hormone-independent neoplasms, if one imagines the latter ef-fects being mediated by other normal somatic systems that are hormonally responsive. Alterations in neoplastic progression and overall clinical status may lead to several important outcomes. First, tumors are capable of producing a variety of "humors" and ectopic hormones and growth factors (Frohman, 1981). Only a small number of these have been identified and in any sense quantified. However, those ectopically produced hormones that have been described are frequently capable of exerting profound biological activity, which not only may alter many somatic systems in the body (for example, tumor-induced hypoglycemia, hypercalcemia, cachexia, and "B symptoms" such as fever) but also may have important effects on psychological functioning. For completely unknown reasons, Hodgkin's disease and non-Hodgkin's lymphomas have a worse prognosis when B symptoms are present, even though, by pathological staging, all other measures of tumor extent are identical. Similarly, for virtually all human malignancies, a poorer performance status is associated with a decreased responsivity to systemic therapy and a diminished survival. Something of a chicken/egg problem contributes to the difficulty of assessing the relative importance of tumor and host contributions. Do tumor humors suppress the immune processes or alter mood and affect, or do alterations in mood and affect occur first and contribute to tumor progression? The answers must await further studies.

As previously mentioned, all tumors capable of growing beyond a mass of a few cells are certainly capable of producing some growth factors. This fact is deduced from the observation that all the stroma and vasculature supporting the tumor are made up of nonmalignant cells that are induced to proliferate by products derived from the tumor. One may readily imagine how hormonal changes could alter a tumor's ability to elaborate such factors without directly affecting tumor growth rate. Such alterations would indirectly alter rates of tumor progression. Since it is likely that most growing neoplasms represent a relatively small positive balance between growing and dying cells, even a small alteration in cell death rate may lead to regression of an otherwise proliferating tumor.

The second way in which alterations in tumor progression may have profound effects on the host has to do with the psychological impact of perception of changes in clinical status and prognosis. Observation of a very limited number of cancer patients is all that is required to appreciate the enormous mood and emotional swings that accompany the delivery of either good or bad news concerning progression or regression of disease. In many instances disease status is not readily perceived by the patient. For example, in the adjuvant setting, patients at high risk of relapse are treated with systemic therapy in order to reduce or eradiate micrometastases. Many other patients have disease that can be followed only by laboratory studies, such as X-ray examinations. These patients are commonly "staged" at predetermined calendar intervals. Patients approach these clinic visits with extraordinarily higher anxiety levels than they approach other routine visits. It is impossible to imagine that the wide emotional swings accompanying reception of significant news concerning disease status will not have a major impact on many body systems.

The difference between a visible skin recurrence of a tumor that commonly metastasizes to skin, such as melanoma or breast cancer, may be no more than a single doubling of the tumor. Approximately 5×10^8 tumor cells represent a half gram of tumor (a palpable lump), and half or a quarter of this will almost assuredly go unnoticed. Yet this tumor has already had to double at least thirty times to reach this size. However, on the day a patient finds that tumor, a day certainly devoid of any significance in the intrinsic progression of the tumor, the most profound emotional response can be unleashed. The patient may at that moment believe that he has crossed from cured to doomed. These perceptions of clinical status and prognosis obviously will substantially alter emotions such as stress, anger, and fear. These enormous emotional forces through previously described mechanisms can lead to accompanying changes in hormonal status.

The impact of the realities of disease status on induced hormonal changes will depend on the extent to which the individual perceives these inputs as different or significant. Individuals capable of appropriately coping with these external stresses may be vastly more successful at preventing hormonally induced changes. Investigators have observed, for instance, that breast cancer patients who are passive and express inappropriate emotions (for example, euphoria in a clinically serious situation) have worse outcome than patients who "feel" the impact of their cancer but respond to it appropriately (Derogatis, Abeloff, and Melisaratos, 1979).

Finally, the chronic psychological status of the individual may play an important role either in facilitating tumor promotion or in dampening or accentuating the impacts of environmental stress. Some depressed patients have abnormal responses to exogenously administered glucocorticoid, and many other endocrine abnormalities have also been described in patients with different psychiatric disturbances (Carroll and others, 1981). While it is beyond the scope of this presentation to review these disturbances, such an altered substrate may greatly change both the ability to perceive external stimuli and the impact of such stimuli on the endocrine status of the individual.

Thus, in summary, it appears highly relevant to study the relationship between various psychological states and tumor progression. The human endocrine system provides one critical mediator of interaction between psyche and tumor. Since virtually all tumors are subject not only to growth regulations but also to alterations in their degree of differentiation and interactions with their environment by changes in their endocrine milieu, it seems inescapable that psychic factors which can evoke such endocrine changes will have effects on actual tumor biology.

7

☒☒☒☒☒☒☒☒☒☒☒☒☒☒

Behavioral Factors
Contributing Directly
to Progression of Cancer

A review of the two preceding chapters—one concerned with central nervous system control over the body's immune apparatus (Chapter Five), the other concerned with hormonal effects on tumor response (Chapter Six)—should suggest that there are multiple, complex mediating pathways linking emotion, cognition, and behavior with the course of at least some subsets of malignancies. One could easily devote a book—or, indeed, several books—to this research area. In this chapter we will review the human and animal evidence for the direct role that behavior may play in cancer risk. The focus will be on factors associated with progression of disease, rather than cause of cancer, because the evidence is much more persuasive in this regard.

The fundamental question that we are asking is: Why is there variance in cancer progression? Why do two patients with identical tumor types, identical stage at diagnosis, identical cellular histology, and identical treatment have different disease outcomes? What proportion of this outcome can be attributed to behavioral and emotional factors? If behavior is a significant biological response modifier affecting tumor course, then this is one source of variance that we may be able to modify. But if we modify the behavioral input, would the course of established malignancy be affected? That is, even if we can show that certain behavioral patterns are associated with specific cancer outcome, this does not necessarily mean that we can modify the disease course by altering the behavioral input. The ultimate answer to the question of "So what?" will finally be obtained after investigators have conducted clinical trials, changing patients' behavior in a randomized treatment group, and looked at outcome effects over and above biological interventions. We are some distance from reaching this last stage of investigation. In the meantime, various case anecdotes of mysterious cancer regression suggest that host characteristics do have some effect on the course of disease.

In Chapter Six, the case of Béla Bartók, the composer, was described. Bartók was dying but rallied in order to complete a new composition for the Boston Symphony Orchestra. He remained alive until the work was complete. A similar kind of story is often told in various works concerned with belief and disease. In the 1950s Krebiozen (a now debunked anticancer drug) was being tested. A particular patient with advanced lymphosarcoma was terminally ill and asked for Krebiozen treatment. Amazingly, he went into remission, returned to work, and resumed his normal course of activities. As published reports began to appear that Krebiozen was worthless, the man immediately relapsed and again became terminally ill. His physician, feeling justified by the dire circumstance, reportedly told him that a special, pure form of Krebiozen was in fact effective, and instead gave his patient distilled water (believing that the earlier rally was a placebo effect). The patient subsequently made a remarkable recovery. Approximately two months later, an authoritative government report on Krebiozen was published; it concluded that the drug was absolutely worthless. The man died a few days later. Finally, Stoll (1979, pp. 24–25) cites the case of a nun with cancer of the pancreas—the diagnosis confirmed by three pathologists. After the other nuns in her order interceded on her behalf with prayers, she grew stronger and returned to work. Seven and a half years later, she died suddenly. "Autopsy revealed a massive pulmonary embolism but positively no evidence of tumor."

Other stories have less felicitous outcomes. For example, cases have been reported of good tumor control and no evidence of disease for years, and then—following a sudden trauma, such as a car accident or a surgical insult—a sudden eruption of the same malignancy (proven the same tumor by biopsy and the histological identity with former disease). We shall return later to the question of tumor dormancy and mechanisms of tumor restraint.

Problems in Human and Animal Studies

Methodological Problems. Studies of behavioral factors contributing to cancer cause are methodologically very difficult to conduct. Therefore, few valid studies exist in the literature. Difficulty arises partly from the fact that, due to cell-doubling time and the indolent nature of these tumors, typically years elapse before tumors are clinically detectable. Therefore, even true prospective studies that follow individuals for significant periods of time may include persons with cancer, misclassified as initially healthy. Behavioral patterns observed in such samples may be in part (undetermined) a result of occult cancers rather than a cause of or contribution to cancer initiation. Even if one were to follow a truly cancer-free sample for many years, the final cancer case yield probably would be quite small. For example, in Thomas's (1983) Precursors Study, where a large number of medical students have been followed for thirty years, only twenty-nine cases of serious malignancy have occurred.

A few provocative studies, however, have been reported. In one relatively recent longitudinal study (Shekelle and others, 1981), 2,020 middle-aged men, employed by Western Electric, were given the Minnesota Multiphasic Personality Inventory (MMPI) at baseline testing and were followed up seventeen years later. The investigators found that—after controlling for age, cigarette smoking, alcohol consumption, family history of cancer, and occupational status—elevated risk for cancer was still significantly associated with high scores on the MMPI Depression subscale. Many other retrospective and mini-prospective (for example, pre- to postdiagnosis) studies and a few other true prospective studies have appeared in the literature. Most of these studies have methodological limits. For example, retrospective studies of personality differences between diagnosed patients and controls reveal differences that are very likely to be the result of having cancer and knowing the diagnosis. No conclusions can be drawn about etiology ten to twenty years earlier. And many mini-prospective studies that follow patients from before to after the diagnosis try to predict disease status on the basis of personality measures given before definitive diagnosis has been made. The results of such studies are likely to be contaminated with clinical "clues" to the true nature of the disease being diagnosed. For example, the physician may express alarm or special concern before definitive laboratory test data are available. Therefore, the patient senses the true nature of his disorder, and statistical findings reflect a link between such knowledge and current disease status. Again, no conclusions about etiology can be drawn from such work. (For a good review of these studies and their limits, see Cox and MacKay, 1982.)

Therefore, little can be said about the role of personality, coping, and emotional factors in human cancer initiation. (Animal studies have measured susceptibility to tumor "take" in transplanted or induced tumor systems as a function of behavioral factors, and these will be considered later.) Clinical evidence for behavioral factors playing a role in progression of disease is much more persuasive.

Requirements for Types of Tumors Studied. If one is going to consider potential effects of behavior, broadly conceived, on tumor course, there are some tumor requirements for study. First, only tumors that have a relatively *indolent course* can be considered. This would rule out the virulent types of cancer, such as pancreatic or primary liver cancer, where it is unlikely that behavioral factors would play much of a contributing role in their outcome. A second tumor requirement is that there must be a rather wide interindividual variation in tumor course, despite similar cell histology, stage of diagnosis, and treatment history. This would allow for some still unexplained disease outcome variance to be potentially accounted for by behavioral and social factors. Third, there should be evidence of hormonal and/or immunological reactivity associated with the tumor in question. Both the endocrine system and the immune system have direct links with the central nervous system; therefore, the probability of finding contributing influences of the host's molar behavior to tumor course is enhanced.

Several different cancers fit these requirements. These include breast cancer, melanoma and other skin cancers, prostatic and endometrial cancers, some leukemias and lymphomas, and colorectal malignancies. Nearly all the clinical studies, few as they are, have been conducted with melanoma and breast cancer patients. The animal studies have used induced and transplanted tumors of various kinds, including transplanted mammary cell lines and chemical induction of mammary and colon tumors.

Problems in Comparing Animal and Human Cancers. In some sense, the clinical studies—complex as they are, considering the organism involved—are easier to interpret than the animal studies—if the human sample is a tightly controlled one and the design is a "clean," prospective investigation. One knows with certainty the cell histology, the tumor type, the treatment, the confounding variables, or the potentially confounding variables, and disease outcome at follow-up within the relevant host of concern—the human organism. On the other hand, animal studies are more difficult to interpret if one wants to generalize to the human condition. First, most animal studies are not concerned with spontaneous tumors, whereas most human tumors are of "spontaneous" origin. Strictly speaking, of course, cancers arising as a result of occupational exposure to carcinogens or skin cancers arising as a function of exposure to excessive solar radiation are induced. The animal studies of such cancers, using *induction* by UV radiation or induction by occupational carcinogens, are directly relevant in this case to the human condition—although the proportional amount of carcinogen required to induce tumors in the animal host usually far exceeds probable exposure levels for humans. The correspondence between animal and human cancer is much more questionable in cases where mammary tumors are induced in animals by the chemical DMBA, since it is doubtful that this human adenocarcinoma is initiated by the same mechanism. Not only is there a difficulty in generalizing from an induced tumor model directly to the behavior of its human counterpart, but even the same transplanted or induced tumors respond differently as a function of experimental animal strain and species.

If one is going to consider the intact animal host as a better system for understanding tumor response than an *in vitro* model, then one would lean more heavily on findings from *in vivo* animal studies. But if, as Henry (1982) points out, the human host is essentially distinct from other species, then one is going to weight most heavily findings from human studies of host response and tumor progression or containment. In the following passage, Henry (1982, p. 378) eloquently captures this distinction:

> The same limbic mechanisms transform social perceptions into neural hormonal responses in mouse and man. The same social bonds of attachment behavior link them, and they are driven by the same need for control of access to food, water, harborage, mate, and dependent young. Mice, no less than men, are capable of changes in the elation-dejection corticoid axis; they, too, can relax and groom themselves. They can also engage in intense fight-flight activity and can be socially successful mates or rejected subordinates. The enormous complexity of human society and man's capacity through his symbol system to identify with more powerful beings (gods or chosen leaders or institutions) give him certain invulnerability to limbic system arousal as long as he perceives himself to be socially supported here or in the hereafter. But if, as the result of early or late experience or a combination of both, he comes to perceive himself as helpless and lacking power to control his state, he may well become more vulnerable than an animal whose associational cortex is more limited.

Man and mouse differ in fundamental ways. Most notably, man has the capacity to symbolize, to project future situations in fantasy, and to resensitize himself continually in reaction to real or imagined stress conditions—so that, for example, the notion of "acute" versus "chronic" stress, an important distinction in animal studies, does not so neatly hold for the human condition.

Breast Cancer Studies

As indicated earlier, the two tumors that have been the focus of human studies in this area are breast cancer and melanoma. Since my own area of investigation has been breast cancer and factors affecting tumor progression, a discussion of this cancer might be pertinent here.

Breast cancer is the leading killer of women dying of malignancy. In 1980, approximately 35,000 women died of this disease. Forty percent of premenopausal breast cancer patients who were diagnosed with three or more axillary lymph nodes containing cancer will have recurrences within five years; only 50 percent of the patients with freely movable nodes and 20 percent of the patients with fixed nodes will be alive ten years after the original treatment. Breast cancer patients who have a disease-free interval (DFI) and then have recurrent disease will live, on the average, fifteen to twenty-four additional months (Henderson and Canellos, 1980).

Host Mechanisms That Control Tumor Growth. The malignant process begins with cellular transformation from normal to neoplastic phenotype and typically ends with progressive proliferation and metastatic spread to vital organs and subsequent death of the organism due to direct or indirect disruption of vital function. In recent years animal research has been carried out to determine restraint mechanisms modifying tumor growth (Wheelock and Robinson, 1983; Wheelock, Weinhold, and Levich, 1981). Tumor dormancy has been defined as the inability of tumor cells to increase in numbers because of some block, which may be positive (for example, immune lysis or destruction) or negative (for example, nutritional deficiency of the tumor bed or supporting tissue structure) in character. Such tumor dormancy is differentiated from the progressive dividing of a slowly growing tumor, which nevertheless proceeds unimpeded. In experimental animal systems, such a distinction is technically demonstrable, for example, by suppressing the host's immune system and stimulating growth of metastatic but quiescent tumors (after surgical removal of the primary) (Wheelock and Robinson, 1983).

In human populations tumor dormancy, while difficult to measure, is at least conceptually consistent with reports of long remissions, followed by recurrence of the same histological type of tumor in the surgical margin (the area immediately adjacent to the surgical incision) following trauma (Wheelock, Weinhold, and Levich, 1981). Indeed, the literature is replete (Stoll, 1982; Everson and Cole, 1966) with clinical examples of histologically identical cells growing from common recurrence sites, sometimes years after treatment.

Wheelock and Robinson (1983) and Yuhus and Tarleton (1978) have linked animal models of tumor dormancy with dramatic human clinical phenomena, such as spontaneous regression of tumors and disease recurrence after intervals of twenty to thirty years. But theoretically we could consider the notion of growth restraint and dormancy when considering the normal clinical course of time from termination of primary treatment to recurrence of disease. Although in humans the measures are not so precise—and factors such as individual cell-doubling time cannot be so readily measured or controlled—still, given the same stage and grade of tumor, we can ask the question: What are the endogenous control mechanisms potentially functioning as restraining agents in the course of this disease?

For breast cancer both *immunological* and *hormonal* mechanisms have been implicated in such tumor growth restraint. Primary breast tumors have been reported to induce an immune response, at last capable of modifying tumor growth, by various mechanisms (Lewison, 1976; Steinhauer, Doyle, Reed, and Kadish, 1982). And a number of studies have shown that hormone levels play an important part in contributing to breast cancer risk, as well as in modulating the course of primary breast cancer, the growth of metastatic foci, and the maintenance of the disease-free interval through endocrine therapy.

Breast Cancer and Hormones. Nearly one hundred years ago, Beatson (1896) noted that an appreciable number of women with breast cancer had regression of tumor when their ovaries were surgically removed. This pioneering work foreshadowed later advances in basic tumor biology and treatment, confirming the importance of endocrine regulation in various tumor systems. (See Chapter Six of this volume.)

Many epidemiologically identified risk factors for breast cancer have a final, common endocrine pathway. Such risk factors include sex (female), age at menarche (younger than twelve), age at menopause (over age fifty-five), age at first birth of a child (over age thirty-five, increasing risk; under age twenty, decreasing risk), and body weight (obesity). Estrogen appears to be a major risk factor associated with a number of these variables, although several different hormones have been shown to modulate breast cancer cells. For example, women who have had their ovaries surgically removed have a decreased lifetime risk of breast cancer proportional to the number of years of menstrual life lost. This protective effect of early castration is lost by the administration of exogenous estrogens. Men treated with estrogens—for example, as treatment for prostatic cancer—have increased risk of breast cancer.

Estrogen receptor status is an important and independent predictor of breast cancer outome (Henderson and Canellos, 1980). Estrogen-receptor-negative (ER-negative) tumors (defined as having less than 10, but as low as at least 3, femtomols of estrodial binding per milligram of cytoplasmic protein) proliferate more rapidly, and patients with ER-negative tumors have shorter disease-free intervals and shorter survival time than those with estrogen-receptor-positive (ER-postive) tumors (Allegra and others, 1979). The positive association between a tumor's estrogen-receptor status and the beneficial treatment effects of adrenalectomy provides support for the notion that the mechanism of action in most patients treated with adrenalectomy is a lowering of plasma estrogen concentrations. In addition to adrenalectomy, antiestrogen drugs, such as Tamoxifen, seem to be effective because they compete for estrogen-binding sites on tumors that are ER positive.

An interesting line of investigation in recent years has been concerned with nocturnal levels of plasma melatonin in breast cancer patients. Normal diurnal variation in melatonin release consists of decreased levels of melatonin during daylight hours and surges of nighttime melatonin release. Results from a series of studies at the National Cancer Institute (Cohen, Chabner, and Lippman, 1978; Tamarkin and others, 1982; Danforth, Tamarkin, Do, and Lippman, 1983) showed altered hormone release curves for breast cancer patients with ER-positive tumors. Patients with hormone-dependent breast cancer have, in fact, a distinctly abnormal twenty-four-hour melatonin rhythm, with a decrease not only in the amplitude of nighttime secretion but also in the total quantity of melatonin secreted. Since melatonin can decrease the number of breast tumors in DMBA-treated rats, and can alter concentration *in vivo* in ovariectomized rats and *in vitro* in human breast cancer cells, the relevance of these findings for cancer risk is obvious.

These investigators also noted that melatonin release may be dependent on sympathetic stimulation of the pineal gland by catecholamines. They concluded that some aspect of this neurochemical signal may be altered in patients with hormone-dependent breast cancer. There is, in fact, a rather large literature indicating that melatonin is synthesized and released from the pineal gland as a function of norepinephrine stimulation (Brownstein, 1975). As will be discussed in more detail later, recent animal models of behavior and tumor response (Anisman and Lapierre, 1980; Weiss, Glazer, Pohorecky, and Miller, 1975; Seligman and Beagley, 1975) suggest that, in animals made behaviorally helpless in the face of stress, norepinephrine (NE) levels in the whole brain and in discrete areas of the brain are depleted—at least during periods of acute stress. Since this model of behavioral helplessness and tumor response is directly relevant to our discussion here, it is important to consider this biochemical link. That is, if NE plays a major role in the release of melatonin, and if plasma melatonin levels are reduced in breast cancer patients, and if this reduced level of melatonin production is strongly associated with ER status and hormonal responsiveness of malignant breast tumors, then one mediating pathway is suggested between behavior and tumor progression.

The puzzle at this point—and it simply underscores that this research needs to be carried out in a single study using humans and not rats—is that this line of evidence, derived mostly from animal studies, would lead one to conclude that melatonin-depleted patients will have the worst prognosis. That is, if melatonin in part affects estrogen levels, and unopposed estrogen is a risk factor in cancer, then patients with reduced melatonin levels—presumably because of depleted norepinephrine-triggered synthesis and release from the pineal gland—should tend to have worse outcome. However, this is not the case. In fact, women with hormone-dependent breast cancer have greater overall survival than patients who lack this receptor protein. The reason for this advantage in hormone-dependent tumor systems remains unclear. Apparently, a major reason is that the treating oncologist can manage these tumors by antiestrogen therapy—that is, by shutting off the excess, unopposed estrogen that feeds these tumor systems. For example, the antiestrogen action by Tamoxifen occurs because this drug competes for estrogen-binding sites on tumors. Nevertheless, if one were to expect the animal model to be relevant to the human condition (and extrapolating from clinical findings related to prognosis and outcome in breast cancer and melanoma patients), one would predict earlier recurrence and shorter survival for the melatonin-suppressed patients. Addressing these links within a human breast cancer sample should help clarify the controlling mechanisms in breast cancer progression.

Breast Cancer and Immune Containment. Many reports have been published on the prognostic significance of lymphocytic infiltration of cancer tissues, including human malignancies (Pross and Baines, 1976; Cochran, 1978; Frost and Kerbel, 1983). The aggregate of experimental and clinical evidence strongly suggests that cellular immune reactions are involved in the host-tumor relationship and play a modifying role related to tumor growth within the organism.

We are not concerned here with tumor immunology in general but with immunological control of beast cancer. There have been reports (Moore and Foote, 1949; Humphrey, Singla, and Volence, 1980) of microscopic studies of *in situ* and invasive breast cancer revealing lymphoid cell infiltrations of the primary tumor. A recent study (Shimokawara and others, 1982) showed that T-cell infiltration in breast tumors was scanty in scirrhus carcinoma but was ample in the infiltrating papillotubular carcinoma, known to have better prognosis. There was also a significant inverse correlation between the intensity of the T-cell infiltration and clinical stage of disease (stage IV having practically no relevant T-cell activity). The intensity of the T-cell infiltration was significantly higher in patients without lymph node metastasis. Although the investigators note that these correlational data do not prove causal effects, they cite animal experiments (Kikuchi, Ishii, Veno, and Koshiba, 1976) demonstrating that some T-cell populations have a suppressive effect for cancer cell growth.

With advancing disease lymphocytic activity decreases—possibly because of the lack of competent, sensitized cells or the lack of tissue antigenicity, or both. One explanation for lack of containment of tumor cells is that those that "slip through" are antigenically modified and thus escape being targeted by sensitized effector cells. It has also been suggested that migrating tumor cells actually lose their antigenic quality and are therefore no longer detected as nonself. (There are other explanations for escape from local control, including the generation of suppressor factors—T cells or macrophages—suppressing immunological containment of tumor cells. Another body of literature is concerned with "blocking factors" in the serum—for example, antigen fractions circulating as antigen-antibody complexes combining with receptor sites on sensitized lymphocytes, blocking tumor cell lysis. These various theories and their supporting evidence will not be considered further here.)

Stage II breast cancer patients have spread of tumor to the regional lymph nodes and, therefore, are presumed to have systemic disease. They typically undergo adjuvant treatment of some form or another in order to kill potential circulating tumor cells before they lodge and grow in different parts of the body. In fact, tumor cells are shed into the circulation in large numbers (Wheelock and Robinson, 1983), and it is surprising that multiple tumors are not seeded at greater rates than they are. The internal milieu is thought to be generally hostile to these new growths in a variety of ways, including destruction by lymphocytes. Stage IV breast cancer patients already have widely disseminated and established tumors, and evidence would suggest that lymphocytic activity plays a minimal role in the control of such tumor burdens.

Naturally Occurring Cytotoxicity and Tumor Control: Implications for Breast Cancer. As indicated above, tumor cells are very adaptive in an immunological environment (shedding antigenic properties, for example), and some populations of heterogeneous tumor mass escape specific T-cell cytolytic attack. In contrast, host cells that kill tumor cells by nonimmune (nonsensitized) mechanisms are effective in killing such heterogeneous masses, including circulating tumor emboli (Hanna and Fidler, 1980). Such nonspecific cells include natural killer (NK) cells and a phagocytic cell, the macrophage. Only NK cells will be discussed here.

NK cells were discovered approximately ten years ago, following the observation that lymphoid cells from healthy volunteers were highly cytotoxic *in vitro* for cultured tumor cells. Since these healthy individuals could not have been exposed to tumor-associated antigen, clearly there was present a naturally occurring mechanism cytotoxic for these cells. Since that time the nature, morphology, and function of NK cells related to cancer surveillance have been intensively studied (Herberman and Ortaldo, 1981).

One major prediction of an immune surveillance theory is that tumor growth should be preceded by depressed immunity. According to Herberman and Santoni (1984), several laboratory and clinical observations are consistent with this theory. In a colony of beige mice having a selective defect in NK activity, a high incidence of lymphomas was found. And patients with Chediak-Higashi syndrome, with a marked and selective defect in NK activity, also have a high incidence of lymphoproliferative diseases. Further, kidney allograft recipients who have received immunosuppressant drugs, and have a high risk of developing lymphomas and other tumors, have significantly lower levels of NK activity (Herberman and Ortaldo, 1981).

Much of the evidence for the role of NK cells *in vivo* has come from studies of transplanted tumor growths correlated with levels of NK cells in the recipient. Most of these studies have shown a strong inverse correlation between levels of NK activity and transplanted tumor clearance. But such evidence does not indicate whether NK cells play a similar role in defense against spontaneous tumors. However, most of the spontaneous mammary tumors in C^3H mice, and spontaneous lymphomas in AKR mice, have detectable susceptibility to NK lysis. In addition, some human leukemias, carcinomas, sarcomas, and melanomas have been significantly lysed with NK cells (Herberman and Ortaldo, 1981).

Therefore, NK cells have spontaneous cytolytic activity against a wide range of tumors, including breast cancer tumors, as well as some normal cells. These lymphocytes have characteristics distinct from other types of lymphocytic cells but are closely associated with large granular lymphocytes, the latter comprising approximately 5 percent of blood or splenic leukocytes.

Direct evidence has been supplied demonstrating that NK cells inhibit tumor metastases *in vivo*. Studies have characterized the role of NK cells in the destruction of circulating sarcoma and melanoma cells (Hanna and Fidler, 1980). Specifically, mice with low NK cell activity—as a result of pretreatment by cyclophosphamide, young developmental age, or congenital deficiency—have a high incidence of experimental tumor metastases. In contrast, metastases in mice whose NK cells are activated by the induction of interferon are markedly inhibited. More recently, systemic adoptive transfer of normal spleen cells to cyclophosphamide-treated recipients twenty-four hours before tumor inoculation reduced the cyclophosphamide-mediated enhancement of pulmonary tumor metastases by transplanted melanoma or sarcoma tumor cells (Hanna and Burton, 1981). Reconstituted cells provided two of the cyclophosphamide-treated animals were demonstrated to be NK cells, as the additon of anti-NK-1.2 antibodies prevented control of metastatic spread. In the *in vivo* model described by Hanna and Burton, the NK cells were most effective during a limited time period (up to twenty-four hours) after tumor inoculation, and the investigators concluded that their target, most likely, was the circulating tumor cell.

While most of the evidence for NK activity against cancer cell spread has been supplied by laboratory, experimental investigation—with limited correlational evidence for an NK role in rare clinical subpopulations, such as patients with Chediak-Higashi (NK-deficient) disorder—other clinical evidence for their role is emerging. According to Steinhauer and associates (Steinhauer, Doyle, Reed, and Kadish, 1982), patients with a variety of advanced cancers (including advanced breast cancer) exhibited lower NK activity against standard target cells (K562) than did patients with localized malignancy or normal controls. NK cells from these advanced patients were normal in number but had reduced functional capacity to kill cancer cell targets. Findings from the study of breast cancer patient prognosis conducted at the National Cancer Institute (Levy and others, 1985) revealed a significant association between NK activity at baseline testing and disease prognosis for these patients. We will consider these findings in further detail in the section headed "Coping and Prognosis for Breast Cancer and Melanoma."

Therefore, based on the large animal literature, as well as emerging clincial evidence, it is becoming increasingly apparent that naturally occurring lymphocyte cytotoxicity may play an important role in controlling the spread of micrometastases within the organism.

The Immune System and the Neuroendocrine System: Implications for Breast Cancer. As we have seen, hormones potentially affecting breast cancer (for example, melatonin, estrogen, and steroids) are modulated by neurochemical (for example, catecholamine) input, and steroid and neuropeptide levels are regulated by hypothalamic, pituitary, and adrenal mechanisms. Similarly, lymphocyte function is modulated by steroidal agents, such as cortisol in man and corticosterone in animals. For example, animals with high corticosterone blood levels show reduced levels of immunoglobulin-secreting cells in the spleen (del Rey, Besedovsky, and Sorkin, 1984); and among the variety of lymphocyte subpopulations modulated by steroidal agents is the natural killer cell—either directly inhibiting NK cytotoxicity or indirectly inhibiting natural cytotoxicity by enhancing suppressor cells, which in turn suppress cytolytic action (Herberman and Santoni, 1984).

In addition, lymphocytes have receptors for neuropeptides (such as met-enkephalin), and they also produce hormonelike substances—for example, lymphokines such as interferon. In fact, Blalock (1984) makes the argument that—because of common peptide signals between the immune system and the central nervous system–endocrine system (for example, ACTH produced by both lymphocytes and the pituitary), common receptors (for example, receptors for neuropeptides on both endocrine and immune tissues), and common function (for example, products of lymphocytes, such as interferon, have hormonelike action)—both the immune system and the central nervous system serve *sensory* functions in the organism. "It [the immune system] has receptors and senses noncognitive stimuli (bacteria, viruses, antigens, and so on) that are not recognized by the central nervous sytem. This information is then relayed to the neuroendocrine system by lymphocyte-derived hormones, and a physiologic change results. Contrariwise, central nervous system recognition of cognitive stimuli results in similar hormonal information being conveyed to and recognized by hormone receptors on lymphocytes, and an immunologic change results. Thus, the two systems actually represent a totally integrated circuit" (p. 1069).

Weber and Pert (1984) speculate about the functional implications of the fact that a network of cells in the brain, glands, and immune system probably communicate via the same chemicals and receptors. They suggest that this "psychoimmunoendocrine network" plays a major role in regulating vertebrate homeostasis. "Much of this network of neuropeptide-secreting cells with neuropeptide cell surface receptors [is] located within the parts of the vertebrate brain which control emotions (limbic system). This raises the exciting possibility that the peptidergic psychoimmunoendocrine network is the biological substrate for mood which constitutes the neural control of the immune system."

Therefore, the modulation of specific cells within the specific psychoimmunoendocrine, homeostatic network may have direct bearing on breast cancer control and metastases, with clearly plausible central nervous system pathways of influence.

Coping and Prognosis for Breast Cancer and Melanoma

Kobasa, Maddi, and Kahn (1982) suggest that hardy individuals are those who have certain personality tendencies—commitment, control, and challenge—that enable them cognitively and behaviorally to manage and adapt to stressful impingement in a way that reduces host vulnerability. And there is evidence that commitment (rather than passivity and avoidance), control (rather than helplessness), and challenge (rather than rigid protection) may play a role in cancer risk. For example, Greer and colleagues (1979, 1985) showed on ten-year follow-up that women who were rated as helpless or stoic had worse breast cancer outcomes than women who were rated as showing a fighting spirit or who denied the significance of their illness. Only tumor grade also predicted breast cancer mortality. A problem with this study is that lymph node status was not part of the survival analysis equation because not all patients underwent axillary node dissection. The authors argue, however, that the prognostic significance of original nodal status decreases after ten years. Certainly there is a consistency between these findings and those of other investigators.

For example, Rogentine and associates (1979) reported significantly greater relapse in melanoma patients who expressed little difficulty adjusting to their disease than in those who reported difficulty in adjustment. This reporting of few problems was interpreted as a passive or stoic response style—an insistence that life would be normal and that they would get on with it. A recent, unpublished prospective study of melanoma patients (Visintainer and Casey, 1984) demonstrated a similar association between passivity and disease course. In this study melanoma patients who reported higher distress, along with a "problem-solving" orientation at baseline, had reduced psychiatric disturbance, higher activity levels of natural killer cells, and less disease relapse nine months later; patients who reported no distress—and no problem-solving orientation at baseline—were more disturbed, had lower levels of NK activity, and higher levels of cancer recurrence at nine months' follow-up. These findings suggest an adaptational process over time and the need to study coping and vulnerability (biological and psychological) as aspects of that process. Similarly, Derogatis, Abeloff, and Melisaratos (1979) reported longer survival in breast cancer patients who were rated as distressed and who reported more psychiatric symptoms of various kinds than in women who appeared to have little psychological difficulty. All these studies have some methodological weaknesses; but, as an aggregate, they show consistent findings: Patients who are characterized as passive have worse cancer outcome.

In a study of coping styles, Jensen (1984) showed more rapid metastatic spread in breast cancer patients associated with a defensive coping style: lower levels of self-reported distress and higher self-report of helplessness, accompanied by symptoms of chronic stress (symptoms of constant tension, inability to relax, and so on). Jensen speculates that inattention to biological signals of distress among individuals identified with a repressive coping style (Schwartz, 1983) might be associated with poorer outcome at follow-up.

Ongoing work at the National Cancer Institute in Bethesda (Levy and others, 1985) and at the University of Pittsburgh School of Medicine has revealed similar patterns of association between a passive, "helpless" response style and worse breast cancer prognosis and outcome. An early pilot study conducted with advanced breast cancer patients (first recurrent patients, with a disease-free interval of at least two months) replicated the findings of Derogatis, Abeloff, and Melisaratos (1979). In general, patients who reported little in the way of psychiatric stress at baseline testing (at the beginning of their treatment for recurrent disease), and who were rated by others as "well adjusted," were more likely to be dead at one-year follow-up. On the other hand, patients who reported higher levels of psychiatric symptoms and were rated as being "disturbed" by observers tended to be alive after one year. These psychological response factors were statistically independent of any biological factor differentiating outcome groups (the only biological factor differentiating outcome groups was in fact the disease-free interval, with a positive correlation between the length of the disease-free interval and survival time). This finding suggests that the psychological factors might be independently contributing to outcome, rather than merely confounded with biological status and hence adding little to outcome variance.

In late 1981 I and my collaborators at the NCI began gathering data on early-stage breast cancer patients. In that study we added the measurement of an immunological mediator—the natural killer cell—and found NK functional activity to have prognostic significance in our sample. When we divided the sample into median NK activity level (NK activity ranged from 8 percent cytolytic activity to 61 percent, median equal to 26 percent target cell lysis), patients who had higher levels of NK activity at the time of primary treatment had significantly fewer nodes positive (mean = .26 nodes positive vs. mean = 2.7 nodes positive, respectively; $F(1, 50)$ = 6.3, p < .01).

Of course, a causal association can be considered only if NK activity is fairly stable over time, and lower functional levels of NK activity presumably precede the spread of tumor cells to the region. Test-retest correlation for NK activity in a subset of these patients (N = 36 over a three-month period) was approximately +.5, p < .003. Therefore, it is certainly possible that lower levels of NK activity preceded diagnosis and were present at the time of regional tumor spread. These data suggest that NK cells are a relevant immunological effector cell in our patient sample.

We then investigated the relative contribution of both clinically and theoretically derived behavioral, psychological, and demographic variables to NK activity at the time of primary treatment by a stepwise multiple regression analysis (Cohen and Cohen, 1975). In general, we found that patients who were rated as "adjusted" by independent observers (that is, who made no complaints and had no apparent psychological difficulties), who complained about a lack of social support from their families, and who responded with a listless, apathetic response style tended to have significantly lower levels of NK activity than patients who appeared more disturbed. These latter patients, while perceiving themselves to be emotionally supported by family and friends, tended to be more negatively reactive at the time of interview. In fact, on the basis of these three factors—observer rating of adjustment, perceived social support, and level of reported listlessness—we could account for 51 percent of the NK variance in these patients.

Results from this ongoing prospective study are consistent with other clinical investigators' findings, as well as with laboratory *in vitro* and *in vivo* data. Suppression of anger and a passive, stoic response style seem to be associated with biological risk sequelae, Recent animal research, which we will further consider in the next section of this chapter, has shown that a passive, stoic response style seem to be associated with biological risk sequelae. Recent animal research, which we will further consider in the next section of this chapter, has shown that pathway to explain the findings related to tumor containment by endogenous host mechanisms.

The effects of *social support* have also been studied in other cancer patient samples, but very few investigators have looked at biological advantage as the end point. And even fewer have looked at possible mediating mechanisms linking social support and host vulnerability. In prospective studies of large community samples, Berkman and Syme (1979) and more recently George Kaplan (personal communication, Nov. 1, 1984) at the Human Population Laboratory in Berkeley, California, showed that intact social support systems were associated with reduction of mortality. Other investigators have studied the effects of various environmental support systems on recovery from breast cancer surgery (Funch and Mettlin, 1982) and on survival from breast cancer (Funch and Marshall, 1983). Funch and Marshall found that social involvement was independently related to survival time. In fact, both stress and social involvement independently accounted for twice as much variance in survival as stage of disease at diagnosis.

In the early-stage breast cancer study discussed above (Levy and others, 1985), perceived social support—the perceived quality of intrafamilial social support—turned out to be significant. Women who complained about a lack of social support in their environment—that is, decreased communication with spouse, poor quality of spousal relationship, and general inadequacy of family social support system—tended also to be in the worst prognostic category. This variable accounted for nearly 15 percent of the NK variance in our sample.

The whole area of social support research has been fraught with methodological difficulties. But the research findings that have emerged, particularly considering the few studies that have examined biological sequelae and host vulnerability as end points, suggest that the quality of perceived social support plays a role in host vulnerability to stress and, hence, disease risk.

Below are two excerpts from breast patient interviews that were conducted as part of the ongoing National Cancer Institute/University of Pittsburgh School of Medicine prospective study. Because of recent animal studies demonstrating an association between behavioral helplessness in the face of uncontrolled stressors and faster tumor growth (Visintainer, Volpicelli, and Seligman, 1982; Shavit and others, 1984; Laudenslager and others, 1983; Greenberg, Dyck, and Sandler, 1984), we used the content analytic strategy of Seligman and colleagues (Peterson, Seligman, and Luborsky, 1983) for extracting causal explanations denoting helpless tendencies from patient interviews. We are beginning to examine the association between such helpless tendencies and breast cancer prognosis in our sample of patients. Patient 1 and Patient 2 were rated as *more* and *less* prone to helplessness in the face of additional stress, respectively.

Patient 1

Doctor: Women with breast cancer have different ideas about what to expect from their cancer. I wonder if you could tell me some of your ideas.

Patient: What I expect in the future?

Doctor: Um-hm.

Patient: Well, I hopefully want to get rid of the cancer cells. That's why I'm going for all of this. That's just my attitude—I just want to get rid of it.

Doctor: Do you have any expectations?

Patient: I expect to do well. I expect the chemotherapy to help me. I know I'm going to suffer some through it, because, you know, everything doesn't come easy. But I feel like it'll be worthwhile.

Doctor: Are you pretty anxious about it?

Patient: Worried about it not . . .

Doctor: No, about the chemotherapy.

Patient: Well, of course—I don't think I'd be normal if I didn't worry about it a little bit. But I just have the feeling that it's going to all be worthwhile, though. I'm sure there will be some side effects that aren't going to be pleasant. I'm almost certain of that.

Doctor: Women like to know different amounts of information about exactly what's wrong with them. Some women like to know all the facts and others are satisfied with not knowing too much. How would you say you are?

Patient: I like to know everything.

Doctor: Um-hm. Can you tell me what you understand factually your particular cancer to be?

Patient: Well, I know that I had a breast tumor that was malignant. The breast was removed, and I know that I need chemotherapy because there is a spread of the cells—all the lymph nodes, five lymph nodes were involved. And it could be, you know, spread even further than they have found. There is no way of actually, you know, saying definitely they haven't spread somewhere else. That's what I understand about it. I know that it's there and I know that I'm just going to try my best to get rid of it.

Doctor: Women also have different ideas about what to expect from the treatment. I think you've already told me some. Do you have any other expectations?

Patient: Oh, I expect to lose my hair and probably nausea and vomiting. I think that's about . . . I understand it.

Doctor: So, in terms of your treatment, you are expecting some bad side effects but you also expect the treatment is going to . . .

Patient: Yes.

Doctor: You had a mastectomy. Are there any other facts about your treatment that you can tell me that you haven't told me already?

Patient: I think that about covers it.

Doctor: When—I'd like to sort of get a time frame. When did you first discover—you felt a lump in your breast?

Patient: I should be ashamed to admit it, but about a year ago. I kept thinking, well, you know, it's nothing. It's really small, way down, and it'll go away. Maybe it's something that goes along with the change of life, menopause, which I have found out it doesn't. You know, that's not true. I just kept thinking—it didn't bother me or anything. It was just a little small lump, it stayed small. Then the past several months when it started getting noticeably larger, it still didn't bother me or anything—no pain, no soreness or anything. So then I decided, you know, I've just got to get this cleared up. I've got to see a doctor and get it off my mind. It had really stayed on my mind.

Doctor: When did you finally decide to go to the doctor?

Patient: It was about the first of March. I knew, you know, all before the holidays, before Thanksgiving and Christmas holidays. I kept saying to myself, "I've just *got* to go to the doctor and have this checked," because, you know, it started really worrying me. Although there wasn't any pain or anything wrong with it. But I just stayed busy and I said to myself, "I'll go tomorrow. I'll go next week." But things like that, you just can't put it off, so finally I went. And I had this intuition that it was something really serious, you know, after it started getting larger. There's an intuition that you have about your own body. And I wasn't really—when they told me that it was malignant, I wasn't really surprised, because it seems like I sort of expected it.

Doctor: So you were sort of putting off finding out the bad news.

Patient: Yeah, the fear, I guess, kept me away as much as anything. That's really stupid, I know.

Doctor: If you were so worried about it, what finally decided you to go to the doctor?

Patient: I just made up my mind and I kept telling myself, "I'm just going to have to go and get this cleared up, because I just feel like it is something serious." And my daughter—I had told her about it so she kept calling about it, too, and she kept saying, "Well, if you don't go to the doctor, I'm going to drive you." So we finally went to the doctor.

Doctor: The two of you went to the doctor. And during that year you mentioned that there were some changes in the size?

Patient: It started getting larger after it was there a long time.

Doctor: During that year were there any very good or very bad things that were taking place in your life? Especially good or especially bad?

Patient: You mean mentally or emotionally?

Doctor: Or things that were, you know, particularly difficult for you?

Patient: Other than the physical . . .

Doctor: Yeah.

Patient: Well, we were having quite a few financial problems, too, during the year, because . . . everything's gone way down [in my husband's line of work].

Doctor: So that was a particularly stressful time?

Patient: It was a stressful time, too, because we were having it bad financially. In fact, we were even having problems meeting our mortgage payment. We were as many as three mortgage payments in arrears, which was really worrisome, along with this other that I was trying to clear up—the lump in my breast. So I guess maybe that's what put it in the background.

Doctor: So you're saying you could sort of not pay that much attention to your breast because . . .

Patient: There were so many other worries, and, too, my husband and I were—I think it was the financial problems that were causing our problems in getting along with each other. You know, where everything tends to irritate you more and you argue more. So there was quite a bit going on. If everything else had been going smoothly I would have probably sought medical attention sooner, you know, if I didn't have any other worries.

Doctor: So the idea of adding one more . . .

Patient: That was just it, I think.

Doctor: Let's switch gears now a little bit and go to your family. You have one child at home.

Patient: Um-hm.

Doctor: And your husband is at home.

Patient: Um-hm.

Doctor: How would you describe your relationship with your husband now?

Patient: Well, it seems like since this has come up everything has changed. As I say, we were arguing and everything, financial problems last year. But since this has come up, I could not have a more understanding husband. Everything has just switched completely around. I think he's sorry, you know, for things that maybe he said, and I'm sorry for things that I said, and it's just switched completely around now.

Doctor: How is he being right now in terms of support for you? Is he here with you now?

Patient: He's not here right now. He's at home working. But there's no one could be more understanding than he is.

Doctor: Has he come . . .

Patient: Oh, yes, he's been here every day except for one. We only live about 60 miles from here.

Doctor: Did he know about the lump in your breast?

Patient: Yes, he knew about it, but he sort of shrugged it aside. Men just don't seem to understand these things the way women do. You know, they're not well read up on it, or they don't know that much about it. So I think he was really expecting it, too, because there before I went to the doctor I made him more aware of it. And it seemed like—this is really terrible to say, I guess, but it seems like I was so angry at him sometimes that—like I was trying to punish him with this coming up for the way he had treated me for the past year, that I was going to punish him by bringing this up and getting treatment for it and everything.

This patient was rated as "helpless" by this content analytic method because a large proportion of her causal explanations, for negative events especially, were considered internal, stable, and global. That is, she located the source of her difficulties as lying within herself ("I guess maybe [because of financial problems] I put it [the lump] in the background"); as relatively permanent ("I'm just going to have to go and get this cleared up because I just feel like it is something serious"); and as having wide-ranging repercussions ("Everything has just switched completely around. I think [my husband is] sorry, you know, for things that maybe he said").

This patient's perception of her world and of the causes of negative events that occur to her is in contrast with the next patient's views.

Patient 2

Doctor: Women with breast cancer have different ideas about what to expect from their cancer. What are some of your ideas?

Patient: Well, it just was surprising that I had one, because I really didn't have—I never did suffer or anything. Well, that's usual, you do have like a muscle, like, in your breast at all times. And when this one came up a few Sundays ago, sort of a knot, . . . I woke up and it felt like a . . . , like you wake up and find a boil itching and looks like when a boil is filling up to burst. I felt it at evening, and then the next morning I called my daughter and I told her, "Oh, my breast has been itching, this and that. Feels like a boil or an abscess or something." And I told her, and she said, "Well, go to a doctor." I was going to the doctor for my leg, because I had a torn muscle before in my leg, and so instead of going to this doctor this morning I'll go on to the next doctor. And I went on and he told me that it seemed like a little tumor was coming and he wanted me to see another doctor at 3 o'clock. So I went to the doctor at 3 o'clock and he's sitting on the side of the table like this and he pressed my breast and he pressed down and told me he felt a little lump in there and he told me it could be cancer. He said, "I want to put you in the hospital on Wednesday, and Friday I want you to . . . " Like that, you know. I said, "Wednesday?" He said, "Yeah." After I got into the hospital, before he had taken the blood test or anything, he talked about taking the breast off just like that. He said, "Have you made up your mind? Are you going to be operated on?"

Doctor: He hadn't done a biopsy on this point?

Patient: No, he hadn't. And he said, "Your other breast is perfect. Nothing wrong with it." So after I talked to my son he said, "Well, don't let nobody just cut on you like that till he examines you or takes X rays, or anything." Because neither one of them had had any X rays or anything. So I coped with that for a while and said, "Well, I'll go and see what they're going to do." Wednesday morning they called me up and told me to be at the hospital at 3:00. I went. I didn't go at 3:00. I said, "There's nothing they can do to me today." I thought I'd come in around 5:00, you know, and just overnight they'd maybe not let you have anything till next morning. X rays and things like that. I told my husband I'd be home when he'd come because I knew I didn't have to come in till Wednesday afternoon. Well, she says, "Well, 3:00 would be about the right time." I said, "What about 4:30 to 5 o'clock." She said, "Oh, well, anyway before 6:00." So I coped with that. So I was doing my washing, trying to get my children's clothes and everything together, you know. I knew what time I had to be there later in the afternoon, and I wanted to put up all my clothes, get my boys' pants all ironed so everything would be clean. And by 1 o'clock she [the nurse] called me and wanted to admit me into the hospital. So when I went all I had to do was go in, because she had already called. He [the doctor] asked me did I talk to my son. I told them, "Yeah." He said, "Well, what did your son say?" I said, "He asked me whether I was ready to be operated on and I told him I hadn't made up my mind." He said, "Well, you might

as well just take the operation. It's going to be you suffering and not me." But he hadn't done the biopsy yet.
So I said, "Well, doctor, take a look at me. I'm not
nobody's bad patient. I'm not trying to be funny or anything. But my mind is just kind of—won't you let me go
home for a day or so, just where I can concentrate." "You
can go home now if you're not going to take the operation. It's going to be you suffering, and I don't give you
six months if you don't take it tomorrow morning. Ain't
that scary?" And I said, "No, that's not scary. I'll pray."
But I told him, "I can't go home tonight. It's too late.
I don't have no transportation." Friday morning came,
they sent the stretcher to the bed. They came to get me.
No signing, no nothing. Not even a shot or nothing. The
nurse said, "You going with us?" I said, "No, I haven't
had anything," which I hadn't. About 9 o'clock, here they
come again with the prep stuff. I said, "I sent the stretcher away." . . . I said, "Well, if you feel like you want
to prep, go ahead." So they did. "Maybe later on you'll
make up your mind." I said, "Well, that's pushing it
too far." You see, I was getting my mind upset, and my
pressure went up and I got a fever, you know, ain't good
for me, pushing like that, because my mind didn't have
time to do nothing.

Doctor: Sounds like a terrible experience.

Patient: My children will tell you, my flesh like this was quiver-
ing, you know. So my son called me and told me, "Mama,
I'm going to send you tickets. I'm going to send you to
the best . . . in the world. You can stay with me, you
know, be in the hospital and stay over there for as long
as . . . " and I came over here and I've been treated real
nice.

This patient's tone clearly conveys a nonhelpless stance
in dealing with her hospital situation. Her causal assumptions
for negative events in this case were rated as relatively external
("I didn't go [into the hospital at three o'clock because] there's
nothing they can do to me today"); unstable ("My pressure

went up [because] my mind didn't have time to do nothing'');
and discrete, without wide-ranging effects ("I can't go home
tonight [because] I don't have no transportation"). When we
contrast the two excerpts for patients 1 and 2, the general impression conveyed from the first patient is that her sense of herself
is causing wide-ranging negative events in her life; for the second
patient, the general impression conveyed is her sense of herself
as in control of things going her way, and attributing limited
and discrete repercussions from negative events caused by others.

Summary of Clinical Findings

Decades of clinical lore indicating that passive patients
fare worse, early empirical studies, and more recent rigorous
clinical investigations, including the direct and indirect evidence
for mediating immunological and hormonal pathways, suggest
that a passive, stoic response style in human patient populations, at least breast cancer and melanoma populations, is associated with worse cancer outcome. Of course, these findings are
correlational. We cannot make any statement regarding direction of causation. However, recent animal studies using an
analogue or behavioral model of human helplessness have demonstrated a causal effect between tumor course and behavior
within a stress context.

Animal Studies on Behavioral Helplessness

For years there have been studies of variously defined
stress, primarily physical stressors of one form or another, and
tumor growth. (See Levy, 1982; Stoll, 1979; and Chapter Five
in this volume for further discussion of this work.) Many of these
studies have suggested the important role of steroids in mediating
such responses. Recently evidence has emerged demonstrating
that such effects are the result of behavioral *response* to the stress
rather than mere exposure to the stressors. Predictability of aversive stimuli or control over such stressors can markedly reduce
the stressful effects (for example, elevated corticosterone or immune suppression) of such conditions. For example, rats able

to terminate shock by lever pressing demonstrated less severe physiological sequelae (gastric lesions, weight loss) than yoked partners who could not terminate the stressors. Both groups of animals, nevertheless, received identical shock stress.

Numerous investigators have used this yoked, "helpless" paradigm to examine the physiological effects of lack of behavioral control over stressors. In general, animals exposed to such uncontrollable (and acute) stress conditions have depleted brain norepinephrine levels, as well as depleted dopamine and serotonin levels in some brain areas. The extent and duration of such effects vary as a function of age, strain of animals, and social housing conditions (Sklar and Anisman, 1981). Short-term behavioral effects of such uncontrollable experience include the inability to learn and perform complex tasks; long-term effects include sensitization and perhaps conditioning of amine changes. That is, reexposure to the originally uncontrolled stressor (or the cues associated with the stressor) may result in the reinduction of the neurochemical events associated with the original trauma. Such conditioned biological sequelae may profoundly influence subsequent behavior, as a result of the neurochemical disruption, and may make the organism chronically vulnerable to disease processes through, for example, suppression of immune response by hormone activation.

As indicated earlier, a series of studies reported since 1982 from three separate laboratories (Laudenslager and others, 1983; Shavit and others, 1984; Greenberg, Dyck, and Sandler, 1984), suggest a causal relationship between acute behavioral helplessness in rat and mice systems, suppression of lymphocyte function, and faster tumor growth. This relationship seems to be modulated by endogenous opioids, since the experimental effects were reversed when an opioid antagonist was injected. These investigators also examined NK activity in the modulation of NK-specific tumors (YAC-1.3 and SL2-5 NK-sensitive lymphoma cell lines). Shavit and colleagues also tested *in vivo* development and elimination of implanted mammary tumors in female rats.

There are currently at least two controversies in this area of investigation. One controversy concerns the specific endogenous opioids that might be playing a role in lymphocyte modulation. Greenberg, Dyck, and Sandler (1984) spoke of beta endorphin as the peptide of action in their study; however, when one considers the peripheral surveillance of NK cells, it seems much more likely that the enkephalins, being more widely distributed than the endorphins, are playing a significant, biologically relevant role here. Many peripheral nerves contain enkephalins; specifically, the high concentration in the adrenal medulla makes enkephalins a likely candidate for study in the area of coping, helplessness, and tumor response (Cox, 1982).

The second controversy concerns the role of opioids—that is, whether they enhance or inhibit NK activity. Shavit and colleagues (1984) suggest that elevated opioids suppress NK activity, and two recent studies have reported a suppression of tumor growth with the injection of opioid antagonists (Aylsworth, Hodson, and Meites, 1979; Zagon and McLaughlin, 1981). Others have reported opposite effects of opioid activity—that is, lymphocyte enhancement (Mathews, Froelich, Sibbitt, and Bankhurst, 1983; Miller, Murgo, and Plotnikoff, 1984). If one puts more weight on *in vivo* evidence, then one might lean toward the possibility that opioids play a suppressive role in natural immunity, since most of the evidence suggesting that possiblity has been derived from examinations of tumor clearance in intact systems. If we consider the host as a dynamic interplay of systems that function together in a homeostatic network, *in vivo* models may be more appropriate to consider. Relevant in this regard is work reported by Miczek and Thompson (1984), which shows a direct link between *victim* behavior and opioid-like analgesia. Victimized, "helpless" behavior in animals exposed to predator bites was more effective in eliciting an analgesic response than objective number of bites received. Such behavior also proved to be a potent elicitor of analgesia in situations where the animal *perceived* itself as biologically vulnerable.

Therefore, the weight of the evidence in animals strongly suggests that helpless behavior—at least in the acute condition (for humans, it is hard to make a distinction between acute and chronic)— causes faster tumor growth and is probably mediated by lymphocyte suppression, including NK suppression. These effects are probably modulated by endogenous opioids and other stress-related hormones (for example, steroids). Lack of perceived control as a biologically significant form of stress may trigger this vulnerability.

Several investigators have shown physiological "stress effects" when animals, primarily primates, are robbed of their accustomed social support systems. In one such study (Coe and Levine, 1981), an infant monkey was separated from its mother and then was either placed alone in a new environment, permitted to remain in the home cage with familiar conspecifics, or placed in a similar cage with unfamiliar mothers and infants. The typical pituitary-adrenal stress response to separation was reduced only in the presence of the familiar social environment. Others (Laudenslager and Reite, 1984) have also demonstrated such findings.

A recent study by Coe, Wiener, Rosenberg, and Levine (1985) showed a dissociation between behavioral response and physiological indices of distress. The primates who failed to develop major behavioral "despair" responses to peer separations still showed a "distressed" physiological pattern of response. Such a dissociation between observable distress behavior and physiological distress markers may provide a clue to host vulnerability seen in human subjects who appear "adjusted" but have the worst biological outcome (Visintainer and Casey, 1984; Levy and others, 1985).

Therefore, intact social support systems may play a buffering role against the stress produced by a sense of helplessness. Laudenslager and Reite (1984) specifically link the two phenomena by suggesting that the intact social group may provide, through information and group-supported expectation, a sense of control over life stressors.

Behavioral Implications

All the work discussed in this chapter—clinical as well as animal laboratory investigations—is investigatory in nature. The limits are obvious: In clinical studies, only associations have been reported. In animal studies, many tumor models are more or less remote from the human condition. Although the aggregate of findings gives us confidence in specifying the nature and character of behavioral risk factors associated with poor tumor response—one characterized as passive, repressive, and stoic—nevertheless, these studies are under way, and certainly no clinical advice or patient prescription can be given at this point.

However, a thought for consideration: While it is certainly easier for families, nurses, and physicians to deal with a smiling face, this may not be the most adaptive response on the part of the patient in an objectively difficult and dangerous situation. Instead, the expression of complaint—the articulation of distress—may be psychologically adaptive and may even have survival value. Do our medical care environments foster passivity?

A final note: When we consider behavioral patterns associated with, and potentially contributing to, biological end points, we may have to redefine what is psychologically healthy and what is not. That is, patterns of behavior associated with better cancer outcome may be, by common psychiatric definition, pathological. At the very least, we may have to suspend our a priori assumptions about what is psychologically healthy and what is not in such populations.

8

❊❊❊❊❊❊❊❊❊❊❊❊

Conclusion:
Behavioral Implications
for Decreasing Cancer Risk

Approximately 30 out of 220 manuscript pages in this book have been concerned with behavioral implications. Even on those pages, many of the implications drawn were tentative and qualified. Some were not. Temperance in drinking, sun exposure, and sexual activity (in contrast with promiscuous coupling with multiple partners) and cessation of tobacco use—particularly tobacco smoking—seem wise as cancer avoidance strategies. The evidence is fairly good that excessive alcohol consumption (particularly when coupled with tobacco use), excessive and chronic overexposure to ultraviolet radiation, multiple and early sexual partners, and obesity are all contributors at least to some forms of cancer. And since some cancers (for example, many melanoma, colorectal, lung, liver, and esophageal cancers) virtually cannot be cured by current treatments, primary prevention of disease is the best line of defense.

Certainly, individuals who fall within epidemiologically identified high-risk populations should scrupulously adhere to relatively frequent monitoring programs—particularly for sites where some reasonably effective treatment is available for early

disease. And once any individual—high risk or not—is symptomatic, prompt reporting for diagnostic assessment in early
treatment is the only course to take.

Reflecting on the content of this work—particularly the
first half of the book, concerned with direct and indirect behavioral contributors to cancer initiation (Chapters Two and Three)
and indirect behavioral contributions to cancer progression
(Chapter Four)—one gets the sense that following the golden
mean and exercising prudence in one's discretionary behaviors
are cancer protective. But if we do nothing more than "follow
grandma's advice," at least we will have some understanding
of mechanisms involved in the link between behaviors, cellular
transformation, and tumor progression.

Risk Factors and Implications

In this chapter, I will summarize the behavioral implications that we have drawn throughout the chapters and will consider more broadly a place for this topic in the larger societal
picture.

Skin Cancer and Exposure to Ultraviolet Radiation. "Sunbathing
in frivolous pursuit of tanning goes on unabated" (Bennett and
Robins, 1977, p. 205). "[We need a] culture revolution of sorts
with emphasis on the joys of sunrise swimming and twilight tennis, and acceptance of a fair complexion as beautiful" (Poh-
Fitzpatrick, 1977, p. 202), rather than as merely pasty! As we
pointed out in Chapter Two, not all tanning is bad—for those
who can tan. Since sunlight is ubiquitous, tanning provides
a natural shield against its harmful effects. But prolonged exposure, particularly in high-risk, fair-skinned groups—either
chronic or episodic exposure during holidays and weekends—
should be scrupulously avoided, as should frequenting of tanning parlors and the like. Public health programs should be
developed to educate school-age children, especially at junior
high and high school levels, about the various forms of skin
cancers and the profile of particularly susceptible subgroups,
and to encourage changed behavioral habits of twilight swims
and changed perceptions of paleness as attractive. High-risk

teenagers could be encouraged to wear protective screens on a daily basis; and the effectiveness of such intervention programs could be evaluated, since behavior and habits would be the endpoint target to evaluate, rather than incidence of cancer or mortality twenty to thirty years hence. Perhaps because my own son is in the high-risk group (red hair, blue eyes, fair skin that does not tan), I am particularly sensitive to the need to educate the very young in such preventive, protective behaviors. It seems prudent to me, it seems doable, and such a course of action rests on a fairly firm foundation of knowledge concerning radiation effect on skin tissue.

Lung, Oral, and Esophageal Cancer and Exposure to Tobacco and Alcohol. As noted in Chapter Two, tobacco and alcohol consumption takes place within a social matrix and is affected by social expectancies. I suggested that perhaps we are our brothers' keepers at all levels of involvement—from role model as parent to hostess providing party libations. A special burden is placed on trained health care providers. Should they remain passive bystanders, watching patients increase their risk for cancer by continuing harmful discretionary recreational habits? I am not recommending a Big Brother society. This issue is invariably raised in discussions such as these, and behavioral interference is always resisted at some level in Western society. One can do only so much, say those who oppose intervention; if individuals wish to kill themselves, so be it. On the other hand, society pays—directly and indirectly—from such courses of action. Loss of income, loss of productive years from civilization, loss of child care when the parent dies, increased cost of medicine as chronic illnesses take their expensive toll—all follow from discretionary personal habits that increase preventive and unnecessary morbidity and mortality.

Weighing all these factors, health care providers can actively assume a disease prevention orientation, inquiring about levels of alcohol and tobacco consumption on the part of their patients. As Lichtenstein and Danaher (1976) suggest, they can provide information about risk, refer patients to specialized treatment programs, and themselves provide specialized strategies (for example, specific quit date, dietary plans, a "buddy" for follow-up help). Dentists, family practitioners, and nurses see many thousands of people every year who could be helped by a modest investment of time. Although "chair time" for the dentist and "office time" for the physician have not typically been devoted to such preventive activities, there is every reason to suspect that such a reorientation of health care providers would have eventual payoff in reduction of chronic disease.

A variety of cancers—lung and other forms—are linked with exposure to carcinogens in the workplace. Smoking, of course, increases risk in workers exposed to other potentially carcinogenic agents. Although certain behaviors—from tobacco use, to protective behaviors and work practices, to machinery maintenance—lie specifically within the province of the individual worker, management is equally responsible for providing a safe environment, as free as possible from carcinogenic exposure.

In the area of occupational cancer, health care providers have a responsibility to record work history, especially the two longest-held jobs, when cancer is diagnosed. They should record not only the type of occupation but also the specific job duties and specific agents to which the worker was exposed during work practice. Cole (1977) describes the astute clinician as still the individual on the front line of identification of health hazards. However, Doll and Peto (1981) caution that, given the cell-doubling time involved in most cancers, cancer-causing agents in the work environment twenty years ago may no longer be there. Instead, new agents have been developed and are in use, with unknown cancer-causing potential that will need to be tracked in the future. Still, an "index of suspicion on the part of the physician," as Cole refers to it, will facilitate drawing links between increased cancer incidence for population subgroups in various geographical locales and potential causative agents to which such individuals were previously exposed.

For the behavioral scientist, such a link will also suggest explanatory behavioral risk variables that could be modified by future intervention. For example, if a current cancer map depicts a high incidence of bladder cancer in an industrialized section of a state, and if the alert clinicians diagnosing these cancers systematically question the individuals about their work history, increased relative risks might be traced to a particular industry and to particular chemicals used by individuals performing specific line duties in the manufacturing process.

But further than that, the link between exposure and cancer incidence could be refined to include specific work practices and host characteristics of exposed workers. It is only in the development of this last link that a complete risk picture can be developed and points of intervention targeted to reduce risk. One point of intervention is the work environment itself and the development of engineering devices that protect workers. The other target of intervention is the workers themselves—to educate and enhance protective behavior and thus alter an additional causal or contributive pathway to cancer incidence.

Cervical Cancer, AIDS, and Exposure to Transforming Agents. As we saw in Chapter Three, the viral evidence for cervical cancer and for acquired immune deficiency syndrome suggests an infective basis for these disorders. There has also emerged a risk profile for individuals who tend to develop these sexually related diseases: sexually hyperactive, with multiple partners, beginning early in life. We know most about early detection, treatment, and cure for cervical cancer. Young, sexually active teenagers, and women who remain outside the health care system (the disadvantaged, largely poor minorities), are prime targets for educational programs and both outreach and inreach activities. The latter strategy is particularly appealing. A high proportion of the poor find their way into acute-care outpatient clinics and hospital emergency rooms. Aggressive educational and screening programs could be developed in these facilities at minimal expense to provide cancer screening and early detection for such patients. Clearly, this strategy presupposes medical care systems that have built into them provisions for care and follow-up of such patient populations.

Also in Chapter Three, we discussed potential risk factors contributing to acquired immune deficiency syndrome, sometimes accompanied by Kaposi's sarcoma. This is such a rapidly developing area of investigation that our knowledge base regarding this disorder will undoubtedly have expanded by the time this book goes to press. But much of the current research points to a viral basis and a weakened immune system as the end result. Sperm as an allogeneic agent eliciting antibody response is thought to play a role in immune disregulation; therefore, multiple sexual partners over long periods of time may contribute to risk of AIDS. Here again—given the strong evidence for viral contribution in sexually associated cancers—the golden mean, moderation, is probably sound interim advice.

Cancer and Malnutrition; Colon and Breast Cancer and Diet. In Chapter Three we considered dietary risk from a couple of different angles. *Too little*, in a sense, is as serious as *too much*. That is, at an extreme, malnourishment in the disadvantaged and cachexia in a cancer patient can obviously contribute to host vulnerability. Malnutrition contributes to immune suppression, perhaps increased cancer incidence, at least indirectly, and increased mortality due to wasting and inability to tolerate aggressive cancer treatments. Therefore, public health efforts should be increased to feed the malnourished in order to prevent disease, including some cancers, from developing. And continued efforts should be made to develop appropriate technology to maintain the nutritional intake of severely ill patients undergoing treatment—pediatric as well as adult patients. Although evidence has not been forthcoming that such techniques as hyperalimentation to maintain the caloric intake of seriously ill cancer patients increases overall survival, at the very least a better quality of life is retained longer in such populations.

On the other end of the eating spectrum, colon and breast cancer risk seems to be enhanced by excessive caloric consumption, particularly in the form of dietary fat, and colon cancer may be reduced by increased consumption of fiber. Based on the aggregate of what we already know from epidemiological and laboratory investigations, despite the fact that the results from ongoing intervention trials are not yet in, it would probably be prudent to reduce dietary fat consumption in a typical American diet by 10 to 15 percent and to ensure adequate daily consumption of dietary fiber. Such a modification should not be too difficult to accomplish, given a well-designed and implemented public education program.

Cervical, Breast, Colorectal, Oral, Prostate, and Testicular Cancer and Early-Detection Efforts. In Chapter Four we reviewed the evidence for screening efficacy of several cancer detection techniques. For the sites listed here, it is undisputably true that early detection does contribute to morbidity and mortality reduction. Of course, for these various sites, cure rate varies. The cure rate approaches 100 percent for cervical cancer when it is diagnosed quite early. (And still some die of this disease in this country today!) For breast cancer the cure rate (or five-year disease-free rate), if a patient has no axillary nodes involved with cancer, is close to 65 percent. If nodes are involved, the rate drops to approximately 40 percent for the same interval. And for colorectal cancer, where there is still no effective treatment except for surgery, early detection is virtually the only hope.

For these sites (except breast), the disadvantaged in our population are again the underscreened and the underserved—and, again, tend to be diagnosed when the cancer is advanced and less curable. There are many obvious reasons why the disadvantaged are outside the health delivery system, but certain system factors that could be changed act as barriers to early detection of cancer in these population subgroups. Such factors as evening clinic hours, provision of transportation and babysitting services, and continuity of care and systematic follow-up from clinics where the poor are seen are obvious aspects of the process that could make a difference in health care delivery to the disadvantaged and better cancer survival in these groups.

As discussed above, a systematic effort could be undertaken in emergency rooms and clinics, with trained personnel who could convey effectively, on an individual basis, the notion of personal risk factors and could link such a patient educational effort with follow-up continuity—for referral or reexamination at appropriate intervals.

Currently the mortality reduction benefit for early detection is limited to the sites noted (breast, cervix, colorectal, prostate, oral, and testicular). But, we also saw in Chapter Three, in all but the most advanced cases, compliance with proven treatments—proven in the sense that they prolong survival if

not provide cure for the cancer—is the optimal behavioral course
to choose. Our discussion of behavioral implications in this regard focused on health care providers, who need to acquaint
themselves with the latest proven technology for enhancing patient compliance. In addition to altering characteristics of the
regimen where possible (for example, decreasing complexity or
minimizing requirements for massive life-style change), health
care providers might consider the use of such techniques as
patient-provider contracts. Across a wide variety of patient
populations, the use of contracts, with built-in rewards for patient success in achieving short-term and long-term goals, and
with explicit review and renewal options as part of the contract
negotiation, has proved to be a powerful device in optimizing
patient cooperation. As orally administered therapeutics are becoming increasingly administered on a chronic, outpatient basis
(for example, Tamoxifen prescribed orally for estrogen-receptor-
positive, postmenopausal breast cancer patients), such considerations become more and more important. Patient characteristics
that can undermine such therapeutic compliance (for example,
forgetfulness in the elderly woman who lives alone) can be taken
into consideration when the contract agreement is made. For
example, part of the contract for such an elderly person might
be the patient's agreement to link ingestion of Tamoxifen with
other daily, habitual behaviors in order to reduce the probability
of forgetting. If family or neighbors are available, enlisting social
supports to reinforce such contractual arrangements can be particularly effective. Certainly, involving patients more explicitly
in the treatment plan process, perhaps including explicit negotiation of rules and procedures, may also enhance a sense of control in the patients and thus militate against their being victims
of inexorable factors outside their control.

   Victim Behavior and Host Vulnerability. This last point leads
into our discussion in Chapters Five, Six, and Seven—particularly Chapter Seven—of behavioral patterns associated with
worse cancer outcome, once the disease is established. Each patient will be unique, and the requirements of each will therefore
be different. Current research findings should play only an *in-
forming role* for the clinician, providing clues for inquiry and

direction. To promote more effective behavior patterns, clinicians might encourage patients to verbalize distress and complaints and to develop a problem-solving orientation and a sense of control over aspects of their lives where this is still possible—always keeping uppermost the individual needs, differences, and uniqueness of each patient—and respecting limits that make such goals imperfectly realizable.

As health care providers, we must ask ourselves how much the medical delivery system itself contributes to passivity, helplessness, and victimization in our patients. I am not the first to raise these issues. For years writers have described ''good patients'' and ''bad patients'' and have noted that the two groups are viewed and managed differently in the health care system. But findings from recent research have begun to link behavioral passivity (often associated with ''good patients'') with biological mediating mechanisms affecting possible tumor response in some host and tumor systems. Therefore, we are no longer considering psychosocial issues and mental health sequelae; we are raising issues of host vulnerability within a perceived environment that affects homeostatic response and, hence, the tumor-host relationship.

All these issues are a matter of current investigation. But they deserve attention and reflection at this point. The host is inseparable from its environment, and we must consider the whole system if we are to understand how the organism fares over time.

The Cancer Experience: The Heart of Our Topic

The whole purpose for writing this text is to increase readers' understanding of cancer—specifically, the potential effects of behavior and the social context on the course of the disease. But the heart of the matter lies with the patient. It is fitting to end this book by listening to firsthand accounts, struggles, and heroics of those who live with this disease.

Patient A

Doctor: Women with breast cancer have different ideas about what to expect from it. I wonder if you could tell me some of your ideas.

Patient: Well, I think the first thing you do is you go through a period of shock. You know, you say "Who, me? I don't believe that!" And then you say "Well, gee, it's got to be so. They wouldn't stand there and tell you that if it wasn't so." And then you think "Well, I'm going to run and hide from it," and then you think "Well, I can't do that because if I do it's going to get worse." But on the whole, I don't know how you would explain it to anyone. You just, when you first are told you have cancer of the breast, you think "Oh my God, why me?" Everybody, a lot of people mentally say "Why me?" OK. Well, I've dealt with cancer off and on all my life, with it being inside the family ring, so the shock wasn't there for me because I've known all along that I had a high cancer risk.

Doctor: Did you have other family members with breast cancer?

Patient: No. None with breast cancer. I would have expected Hodgkin's or leukemia, or anything but breast cancer. I mean, that blew my mind! But I think having dealt with it as much as I have, it wasn't as hard a blow to me as it was for somebody that's never had to deal with cancer, and something that surprised me was that one out of three people come up with cancer.

Doctor: That what?

Patient: When we first came in down here, they, a social worker downstairs, told us that one out of three people comes up with some form of cancer, which was a shock to me. I didn't realize it was that high. But I don't know, as far as how you feel about it, the only thing you can do is say "Well, I've got it. Let's go do something about it."

Doctor: What are your expectations for the future?

Patient: I'll have to keep a closer eye on myself than I have before. I'm going to do everything I can to insure that it does not come back, but there's no guarantees of that. So I'm gonna enjoy life! And like I said, keep a close eye on myself. If it does come back, well then I'll deal with it again. But I'll keep my fingers crossed that it doesn't!

Doctor: Have you gotten the results of your axillary node dissection?

Patient: No. Not yet. That should come in Wednesday.

Doctor: So you still need to know an important piece of information?

Patient: Yes, but my theory is to cross the worst bridge and then if it's not that, you can always walk away slow. So I've already accepted the fact that they're probably positive.

Doctor: So that maybe you'll be pleasantly surprised?

Patient: Right. I mean, you know, this is what I did to my country doctor. I walked in and I told him, "Hey, I've got a knot on my breast." He said, "Oh, gee, that's terrible. Well, we're going to have to do a biopsy on that." Go outside—come back in. "I don't like the looks of that. How long has it been here?" "Well, gee, Doc, what's the worst it can be, cancer?" "What are you doing, crossing bridges before you get to them?" "No, facing facts and then if it isn't, then we're better off than we were to start with because at least I'm not going to fall apart then." I think if you have a tendency to look at the worst side of things, not be a pessimist, not know that that's what its gonna be but look at it and say, "If it is this, then this is what I've got to do in order to counteract it." I think the worst thing you could do in a situation like this is to come unglued. To just fall apart and go into hysterics. I don't mean that you can't cry—that you can't feel mad or hurt or whatever it is you're gonna feel, but to just completely lose sight of everything and pity yourself, I think that is the worst downfall you could have in something like this. So that's the way I look at it. If you run head-on into it and look at the worst and then if you have a pleasant surprise, then you can say, "Whew! I feel so much better!" But its better than to look at the optimistic side, "Oh, it's not going to be cancerous. It's not going to have spread that far, and I know that." And then they come back and say, "Hey, I'm sorry." Then you're going through it all over again. So what I look at is the worst end and—I don't say that it's going to be the worst, but I say if it is the worst, then I can handle it.

Doctor: Women like to know different amounts of information about their cancer. Some like to know all they can; others don't want to know very much. How do you feel?

Patient: Well, right now I'm waiting for all the information to get in before I hit the doctors with a bombardment of questions. I figure until they have the facts they can't tell me. One thing I do know about doctors is that they do not like to speculate. They'll dance around to keep from telling you anything that is a guess. I don't blame them, because their guess might be completely wrong. So until the facts are in, I'm not asking any questions. Once the facts are in . . .

Doctor: There's a lot you want to know.

Patient: Yeah, well, there's quite a lot—they have explained most of it to me. Of course, like the lymph nodes. I would want to know how many or how bad, how far it had spread, how many they took out. But until all the facts are in, I'm willing to wait patiently but I want to know.

Doctor: To this point, can you tell me what you understand about your situation?

Patient: Well, so far, that cancer was in a central place, except for the lymph nodes which we don't about, which were, well, I could feel one once I got up here. Now my doctor didn't find that back home. I understand that I'm going to, of course with the type of surgery, that I have, that I'll have radiation treatment. If the lymph nodes are positive, I'll go through chemotherapy, also. As far as what type of cancer, I don't really know whether it was, you know, the fast type or slow type or whether it was hormone or what—which is one of the questions I am going to ask so I know if another one comes up how quick I need to get somewhere if it turns out to be the same type.

Doctor: You don't remember your diagnosis, or they didn't tell you what?

Patient: Ummm. Wait a minute. I read it. Cystic carcinoma I believe was the way they had it written.

Doctor: Would it have been infiltrating and ductal?

Patient: Yes, that sounds more like it, I believe. I'm not much, I never took Latin or anything like that so . . .

Doctor: It's not the vocabulary that you come across every day.
Patient: Right. It kind of throws you there.
Doctor: What about your expectations from the treatment?
Patient: What do I expect from it? I expect there to be quite a
bit of change. In my appearance, with the type of surgery
I had, yes, I expect there to be a change. And I expect,
at times, I'm going to feel like saying "What am I doing
here, why am I putting myself through this?" But I think
always in the back of my head, I'll know why. Because
the alternative not to do anything is to die. And I definitely
don't want to do that. I enjoy being here. So if I have to,
I'll go through the chemotherapy. I think that one thing,
the main thing that bothers me about chemo, is the loss
of my hair. But as for the radiation treatment, I don't
know that much about it other than what my brother took.
He took cobalt, and, of course, that was with Hodgkin's
and it made him very sick. I don't know whether it was
that or whether it was the combination or . . .
Doctor: What happened to him? Did he die?
Patient: Oh yeah. He died. But at the time Hodgkin's disease
was a very bad thing.

Patient B

Doctor: Speaking of your treatment, let me just ask you: Different people like to know different amounts of information about the treatments that they're receiving. Could
you tell me a little bit about what your understanding is
of what it is that you're taking?
Patient: Anticancer. Kill the cancer cell—kill it, just to kill it. Well,
if it's in me, even if I'm sick, I tell myself in the long run
it'll be better. But . . . and knowing I'm going through all
this crap and getting nowhere, and maybe I should have
never discovered it, and I should have died with it.
Doctor: What do you expect from the treatment? I mean, this
isn't related to what you just said. Your understanding
is that it's going to kill the cancer.
Patient: Right.
Doctor: And even though it makes you sick. And you said you're
taking Cytoxan and Adriamycin?

Patient: Yeah.

Doctor: Okay. So you know what you're taking. What about your—different people expect different things from the treatment. What's your expectancy?

Patient: I don't know anymore. I thought it was going to cure me. In fact, it's just—maybe I'm in the middle of a, you know, crisis or something. At first, you know, it doesn't matter. Now, like the last two times I've come up here it's like—I want to just die.

Doctor: A what's-the-use kind of thing.

Patient: Yeah. I understand what's happening to me. Don't get me wrong. It's just how I feel myself.

Doctor: But your expectancy as far as the treatment is concerned is that it is going to kill the cancer.

Patient: Yeah.

Doctor: And your . . .

Patient: But the more books I read about it—the more I come up here and everything, before, you know, anything—I went through all that and I still haven't been cured and then I had to come back and do it all over again. You think, "Holy cow! I've got to go through all that again and again and again," you know. Losing a breast isn't half—I don't feel like a woman no more.

Doctor: You don't.

Patient: Un-uh. Not at all.

Doctor: I was going to get to that, but . . .

Patient: I know I'm dead. I can't find a job. I can't go swimming. The only thing I can do is sit in the house.

Doctor: That'll pass, you know. You're right, you're sort of in the middle of things and it's easy to lose your—the big picture.

Patient: That's what I'm hoping it is.

Doctor: But you were saying your expectancy initially from the treatment was that it was going to kill the cancer, but now it sounds like you're kind of not sure, or sort of wondering.

Patient: Yeah, you got it.

Doctor: Different people like to know different amounts of information about the disease and about what's actually going on with them. Would you kind of share with me your understanding of the breast cancer and what's happened to you and what the disease is?

Patient: Well, I discovered it myself. I had a lump. Didn't hurt. And I went to my family doctor and he sent me to a surgeon down in Florida and he called me on Friday the 13th and said, "You've got cancer. Be in the hospital on such and such a date." And I had no insurance or nothing, so I called the Cancer Society and that's how we got ahold of Dr.____.

Doctor: Now, you say you discovered the lump yourself. Okay. Think back now a second. What was the length of time between when you discovered the lump and it was diagnosed as cancer? How much time was between there?

Patient: About two weeks.

Doctor: Two weeks from the time you felt the lump and he said, "It's breast cancer." Okay. During that two-week period, was there any sudden change in the symptom—the lump— any increase in size, change in shape . . .

Patient: No.

Doctor: No change in the color of skin, no change?

Patient: No. But I had a feeling—I didn't know, but I just wanted to make sure. And that's what is was.

Doctor: Two weeks—that was pretty fast between discovering it and being diagnosed.

Patient: Yeah.

Doctor: You know, you were sort of telling me your understanding of the breast cancer and what really was going on with you physically. And that's when you started telling me about the lump and so on. Could you kind of, you know, tell me a little bit more as far as your understanding of the breast cancer and what was really going on with you physically?

Patient: Nothing to it. I mean, you either have it or you don't. It's like being a little pregnant. Either you are or you aren't.

Doctor: Yeah, okay.

Patient: It was something I had to take care of, and I took care of it, you know, the best I could.

Doctor: What about your expectancy with respect to the disease? What do you expect?

Patient: What do I expect? I hope to be cured. That's about it. To raise my kid.

Patient C

Patient: I have talked to others who say that age doesn't matter, but I feel different, I think it matters a great deal. I am going to be sixty-eight years old, so I know my whole attitude is far different from what it would have been had I been thirty-eight or forty years old. I know that, because I had a sister who died of breast cancer. So I know some of the proceedings I might go through. I know not having a husband makes a difference. I don't have to answer to anyone except myself. I have a very positive attitude. I'm not afraid at this point. I don't know if there will come a time when I will be afraid. Cancer is an ominous word, we hate to hear it. I felt more concerned about breaking the news to my family than I did about anything else. None of us are young now. [They all have] something wrong with them, and I didn't want to upset their health balance, and emotional reaction can do that. So to me that was the most important thing. I kept it a secret until I knew more about what I was going to do about the problem. They have handled it very nicely. Our attitudes are very positive.

Doctor: You also said before that you don't expect that there is going to be any more except to come in for follow-up treatments. And you feel optimistic.

Patient: They have indicated that it looked good.

Doctor: So you had a clinically negative report; they didn't feel anything.

Patient: That is right.

Doctor: I wonder if you could fill me in a little bit on how you found the lump. You found the lump yourself?

Patient: Yes.

Doctor: How did you find it? When was that? How did you get here?

Patient: Well, the finding date was June 13 or 12. It was a hot night. My apartment is not air conditioned; I live alone.

I was having guests the next day and was very concerned because I have no air conditioning and it had gotten so hot. I had done a lot of cleaning and shopping for the dinner party. I went to bed that night and I was thinking about all the things that should have been done and whether or not I had forgotten something and got up to do something. I was perspiring. I took off my top to wipe myself. As I wiped myself, I felt the lump. My reaction was "Oh no!" But it was there. From then on I made appointments with doctors to have it checked out.

Doctor: When you said that you had felt it and you said, "Oh no," does that mean that you thought something was wrong immediately?

Patient: Yes.

Doctor: So right away you knew something was wrong or different?

Patient: Yes.

Doctor: Did you decide at that point that you were sick, it was a problem, or just different?

Patient: I can't remember deciding that I was sick. I decided that the odds that this was benign were unlikely, because my other benign lumps were premenopausal. I was inclined to develop lumps. It had been sixteen years since my last aspiration. I felt at this age it was very likely that it was something different.

Doctor: Did you decide right away that you would go to the doctor?

Patient: Yes.

Doctor: As soon as you found it, you knew that you would go to someone to see it?

Patient: Yes. In New York I belonged to HIP [the Health Insurance Plan]. It was a strange set of circumstances because my doctor, whom I had been seeing for thirty years, had died a few months ago. He was my family doctor. He was a nice, solid man who was not inclined to overmedicate. My problem was that I was going to do to all new doctors. People who did not know me. I made an appointment. . . . That was a Thursday or Friday, and my appointment was for the Monday morning. I went for the visit cold. He didn't know me and I didn't know him. He asked about the mammography reports. I said that all I knew about it was that they told me they were okay. I had nothing to show him and he did not ask for another mammography. He said he would not try to aspirate because it was disturbed at that time. He suggested that I make an appointment for an operation. I said that I would like to think it over.

Doctor: For a biopsy?

Patient: No for a . . . the way they do it, I imagine, the way I had it done before, is you sign a paper when you go in and they do it all at the same time.

Doctor: So if it is malignant, they go ahead with the mastectomy.

Patient: I would not have known until I had awakened. He didn't want the operation to be delayed. The next morning I made the appointment for July 25, that would have been in two weeks. In the meantime I had told no one. At that point I discussed it with two friends who agreed to help me through it and notify the family. The more I thought about it, the more nervous I became because I was going in alone. Nobody knew me. I had been referred by no one, and nobody knew except these two friends.

Patient D

Doctor: Um-hmm. Do you expect it might come back? Do you expect it won't come back? Do you expect it's gone? What are some of your thoughts?

Patient: I don't have any idea. I mean, last night on the phone I said to my brother, "I know I'm not going to die from this." And he said, "Do you mean that?" And I said, "Yes." And he said, "That thought has been driving me crazy. I could not ask you that." And I said, "I don't think that I'm going to die from this." I have a friend— my forever friend. If everybody is as fortunate as I, they will have a forever friend. At this moment she is taking care of my sixteen year old, which takes a forever friend! And she has this thing. She said, "I have watched you throughout your life." We became friends—real friends— in about fourth or fifth grade. She said, "I have watched

you throughout your life and all the jams that you've gotten yourself into, and I'm just waiting to see. Every other
time you've come out smelling like a rose. How are you
going to pull it off this time? I know you will! But how
are you going to pull it off this time?''

Doctor: So it sounds to me like your friends are saying—your
family, brother—and you are saying that you're going
to get out of this one.

Patient: Oh, yeah. I'll get emotional and everything. When I
first told my son that the mammogram was very suspicious, I was holding him—he's sixteen [years old], he's
ten feet tall, and he's very much a young man. And he
said, ''Mom, what do we do?'' And I said, ''We fight
like hell, and that's it. You're going to see your mother's
true colors come out. I've always been a fighter and I will
fight it and I will lick it.'' And it was a very emotional
scene, because . . . he's a super-nifty kid, and he feels so
about this whole thing and about me that I haven't hid-
den any of it from him. What has happened is that he
has been there with the first crush of the emotion, which
I am sorry for. However, my forever friend is a nurse,
works in critical care, and so she and I talk after the emotional surge has come, and she gets the facts and then
she sits down and interprets for him. But he still has to
hold on to the factualness that they are doing things and
that, you know, it's scary but it's not the end or anything.
I just hope that he will grow from this and not be scared.
I look at my own brother (the one who called me last
night), and he was very, very close to my father when
my father died, and he was sophomore, junior in high
school at the time, and I believe that when my father died
my brother kind of made a subconscious decision not to
care about anyone so much again in his life, because he
was hurt so deeply. I think slowly he's coming out of that
now, but it's been almost twenty years. And I hope that
doesn't happen to . . .

Doctor: It sounds like with your father there was a suddenness
in his . . .

Patient: Well, he was sick. He became ill on the golf course. He

was playing golf with his best friend, who was a surgeon.
And that was on Sunday morning and he was sure it was
indigestion and the surgeon was sure that it was a per-
forated ulcer. They were all a bunch of frightened . . . you
know, the whole gang of them.

Doctor: The point that I'm trying to make is that it sounds like
a very different situation, being a very acute illness . . .

Patient: Um-hm.

Doctor: And probably your brother had no time to, you know,
have any kind of closeness with him, in the flurry of a
week trying to find out what's wrong with him. And it
sounds like you are not pushing your son out at all. You
are sharing everything that's going on.

All these patients are breast cancer patients, because this
has been the area of my own investigation. But in their subjective response to diagnosis and their immediate handling of the
crisis, they probably are not very different from other patients
diagnosed with cancer. There are themes to note. For example, one theme has to do with the interaction of the patient with
her social support network—friends, family members, and referral systems. The report of the older patient (Patient C) about
her elderly siblings all being chronically ill with some disease,
the death of her long-time trusted physician, and the feeling of
community isolation when choices had to be made is a poignant reminder of the plight of the elderly patient in our society.

But all these patients together reflect in a very immediate
way the devastating blow that the diagnosis of cancer deals. They
also demonstrate to various degrees the individual heroics that
patients are capable of in coping with cancer.

We began this book by discussing Susan Sontag's (1978)
comparison between society's response to cancer in this century and its response to tuberculosis in the nineteenth century
and before. When the cause and cure for TB were unknown,
tuberculosis itself was used metaphorically to capture a sense
of mysterious passion that consumes its frequently young victims—characterized dramatically as spent by such passion and
genius. In this century cancer as a disease process remains a

mystery and, hence, has become a culturally and socially derived metaphor for a sense of rot, decay, corruption from within. The Watergate episode became a "cancer on the presidency," bad characters are described as "malignant," and so on. As long as the disease remains uncontrolled, as long as its cause is unknown, as long as its course is not understood, it will remain a metaphor for the mysterious, the capricious—for evil itself.

It is my hope in writing this book that we are one step closer to demystifying cancer as a disease process. For the reader this disease should now be less mysterious. At the very least, cancers should be understood as multiply determined chronic illnesses, with multiple sources of variance in both initiation and progression. One source of such variance may well be the host's behavior.

Human behavior, complex though it is, can be changed. Those who read this book should derive some hope because this biological response modifier is ultimately under our control. While we cannot promise more than we know at this point, at least our future research direction regarding behavior and cancer and our ultimate goals are clear. As stated at the beginning of this book, it is an enterprise worth all the effort.

Glossary

ALLOGENEIC (ALLOGENIC). Having cell types that are not *histo-compatible*. In the area of transplantation biology, individuals of the same species are considered to have allogeneic cell types if the cell surfaces of their tissues express different *antigens*.

ANAPHYLAXIS. An allergic reaction to foreign protein or other substances. The term originally referred to sensitization in laboratory animals injected with a foreign substance, such as horse serum; it now refers also to human reactions. Such an injection renders the individual hypersusceptible to a subsequent injection.

ANAPLASIA (ANAPLASTIC). Primitive cell structure. A loss of specific cell differentiation, a common characteristic of tumor tissue. Anaplastic cells appear haphazard in shape and in orientation to one another.

ANGIOGENESIS. The process by which tumor cells, by releasing a diffusible chemical factor, promote the growth of blood vessels from surrounding tissue into a solid tumor.

ANTIBODY. A protein generated in the blood in response to foreign substances, neutralizing these substances and pro-

Note: Words in italics are defined in separate entries in this glossary.

ducing immunity against them. Antibodies are classified according to their mode of action as agglutinins, bacteriolysins, hemolysins, opsonins, precipitins, and so on.

ANTIGEN. A substance that is capable, under appropriate conditions, of stimulating an immune response and of reacting with specific *antibody* or sensitized T lymphocytes (see *T cells*), or both. Antigens may be particulate substances, such as bacteria or tissue cells; or they may be soluble factors, such as foreign proteins or toxins. Only the portion of the polysaccharide or protein molecule (known as the antigenic determinant) combines with antibody or the specific lymphocyte receptor.

ANTIOXIDANTS. Enzymes that protect cells from oxidative damage. Many mutagens and carcinogens may act through the generation of oxygen radicals, which are considered major contributors to DNA damage. Protective enzymes include small molecules in the diet that act as antioxidative mechanisms and hence as anticarcinogens. Examples are vitamin E (tocopherol), beta carotene, selenium, and dietary ascorbic acid.

AROMATIZATION. Chemical conversion to an aromatic compound.

AUTONOMY (of tumor cells). Relative independence of a malignant cell's development apart from the needs and requirements of the host as a whole.

B CELLS (B lymphocytes) (humoral immunity). Bursa-derived (or Bursa-equivalent-derived) cells in avian and nonavian species. B cells are the precursors of plasma cells that then produce *antibody*.

(BETA)-ADRENERGIC RECEPTORS. Receptors for sympathetic nervous system input. Adrenergic fibers liberate catecholamine at neural synapses when a nerve impulse passes. The term "adrenergic" is used to signify characteristic of, activated by, or secreting epinephrine or other substances with the same or similar activity.

BOMBESIN. A chemical, classified as a *neuropeptide*, that stimulates gastric acid secretion, gallbladder contraction, pancreatic secretion, and relaxation of the common bile duct and duodenal junction. Bombesin is present in both the brain tissue and the gut of man.

CARBOXYHEMOGLOBIN TEST. A test used to determine the presence of carbon monoxide binding to hemoglobin. Such binding is not readily displaced from the hemoglobin molecule, which normally binds with oxygen. This test is commonly used to detect traces of tobacco use in smokers who inhale.

CARCINOMA. A cancerous growth, comprised of epithelial cells, which tends to invade adjacent tissues and spread to distant parts of the body.

CELL-MEDIATED IMMUNITY. Immune reaction in which the participation of *macrophages* and *T cells* is paramount. (See also *B cells*.)

CHEDIAK-HIGASHI SYNDROME. An inherited immune-deficient disorder involving multiple somatic systems, including central nervous system abnormalities, partial albinism, and a high rate of lymphoreticular malignancies. Patients suffering from Chediak-Higashi syndrome are also deficient in *natural killer cell* activity. There is no known treatment other than antibiotic therapy during infections, and prognosis is poor because of progressive neurological deterioration and increasing susceptibility to infections.

CORTICOSTEROID. A substance produced by the adrenal cortex in response to the production and release of corticotrophin hormone by the pituitary gland. These steroids are divided as a function of their major biological activity into two categories: (1) glucocorticoids, influencing fat, protein, and carbohydrate metabolism; and (2) mineralocorticoids, influencing electrolyte and water balance regulation.

CYCLOPHOSPHAMIDE. Potent anticancer drug used in the treatment of breast *carcinoma* and other cancers. Produces nausea, vomiting, hair loss, and myelosuppression.

CYTOLYTIC ACTIVITY. Lymphocytic destruction of antigenic target cells.

CYTOMEGALOVIRUS (salivary gland virus). One of a group of herpes viruses that infect monkeys, rodents, and man, with the production of large cells bearing intranuclear inclusions or multiple constituents of the cell cytoplasm. Infection with cytomegalovirus resembles as a syndrome infectious mononucleosis.

DMBA (dimethylbenz(a)-antracene). A potent carcinogen.

DYSPLASIA. Abnormality of organization, size, and shape of adult cellular structure.

ECTOPIC HORMONES. Hormones secreted from a source not normally associated with such specific hormone production, such as adrenocorticotrophic hormone (ACTH) being produced by lung cancer cells.

ENKEPHALINS (methionine enkephalin and leucine enkephalin). *Neuropeptides* that have potent opiate-like effects and in all likelihood serve as neurotransmittors. Enkephalins are found within the central nervous system and are also widely distributed in the periphery. Centrally, they bind to the same receptor sites as do the opiates.

ESTRADIOL. An estrogen hormone found in the ovaries and placentas of women. Also produced commercially for use in treating estrogen deficiency.

ESTROGEN-RECEPTOR-NEGATIVE TUMORS AND ESTROGEN-RECEPTOR-POSITIVE TUMORS. Tumors are classified as estrogen-receptor-negative or positive as a function of the density of receptors for estrogen on the surface of tumor tissue. For example, breast cancers are defined as estrogen-receptor-negative when they are found to have less than ten (but as low as at least three) femtomols of estradiol binding per milligram of cytoplasmic protein. Such tumors have been demonstrated to proliferate more rapidly, and patients with estrogen-receptor-negative tumors have shorter disease-free intervals and shorter survival time than those with estrogen-receptor-positive tumors.

FECAL OCCULT BLOOD TESTING (Hemoccult test). Test commonly used in the detection of blood in the stool, a sign of
potential colon malignancy. Slides are prepared from samples of fecal material, and chemical tests are performed
in order to detect the presence of hemoglobin in the feces.

FIBROBLAST. A connective tissue cell that differentiates into various forms of fibrous tissue in the body (binding and supporting tissues of all sorts).

GRAFT-VERSUS-HOST DISEASE. The destructive reactions of lymphocytes within a graft (such as a transplanted organ)
against the incompatible tissues of a host (such as an organ
recipient).

GRANULOCYTE. Any cell containing granules, particularly a
leukocyte containing granules in its cytoplasm.

HISTOCOMPATIBLE. Generally refers to tissues sharing *antigens*
such that transplantation becomes possible without eliciting tissue rejection by host immune reaction.

HTLV-III (human T-cell leukemia virus). A virus that has been
found to be associated causally with acquired immune
deficiency syndrome. Human T-cell leukemia-lymphoma
viruses are a family of T lymphotrophic *retroviruses* strongly
associated with adult T-cell leukemia. A high proportion
of patients with acquired immune deficiency syndrome
also have *antibodies* that react with *antigens* on the surface
of human T-cell leukemia virus-producing transformed
human T cells.

HUMORAL IMMUNITY. See *B cells*.

HYPERALIMENTATION. Administration of more than optimal
amounts of nutrients. Intravenously administered, nutrients are infused into a patient by way of a central venous
catheter (total parenteral nutrition).

HYPOPHYSECTOMY. Surgical removal of the pituitary gland.

IATROGENIC. Generally refers to disorders caused by medical or
other treatment—for example, a case of endometrial cancer
developing as a result of chronic use of exogenous estrogen.

IMMUNE SURVEILLANCE. The notion that the immune system, particularly cells contributing to natural immunity (*natural killer cells*) and *macrophages*, attacks and destroys early cancer cells before such malignancy has an opportunity to grow and spread.

IMMUNOCOMPETENT CELLS. Lymphocytes that have the capacity to respond antigenically to foreign proteins and to develop a "memory" for such foreign proteins. Upon subsequent exposure to these *antigens*, the cells are able to mount efficiently an immune reaction based on previous exposure.

IMMUNOGLOBULINS. Proteins found in the serum and in other body fluids and tissues (including urine, spinal fluid, lymph nodes, and spleen). They are synthesized by lymphocytes and plasma cells and function as specific *antibodies* responsible for humoral immunity (see *B cells*). There are five classes of immunoglobulins: IgA, IgD, IgE, IgG, and IgM.

IN SITU TUMORS. Tumors that have invaded the local tissue but have not spread beyond this tissue of origin to adjacent or distant regions of the body.

INVASIVE TUMORS. Tumors that have spread beyond the original local site to adjacent tissue and, ultimately, to distant organs.

LATENT PERIOD (for tumor development). Period between initial transformation from normal to malignant cell and the time when cancer is first able to be detected clinically. There are differential latent periods for tumors, depending on the cell-doubling time characteristic of the transformed cell involved in the developing malignancy.

LEUKOCYTES. White blood cells. The varieties of leukocytes may be classified into two main categories: granular and nongranular leukocytes.

LYMPHADENOPATHY. Regional lymph node enlargement frequently associated with spread of cancer to adjacent tissue.

LYMPHOKINE. A generic term for soluble protein mediators released by stimulated lymphocytes on contact with *antigen*.

Lymphokines play a role in further lymphocyte transformation, *macrophage* activation, and *cell-mediated immunity*.

LYMPHOPENIA. Reduction in the proportion of lymphocytes in the blood.

LYSIS. Destruction or decomposition of target cells.

MACROPHAGES. Phagocytic cells that originate from bone marrow monocytes and perform numerous accessory functions in cellular immune reaction.

MELANOCYTES. Cells of the epidermis that synthesize the pigment melanin within their melanosomes.

MELATONIN. A hormone synthesized by the pineal gland, which, among other functions, influences estrus in mammals. Its secretion varies diurnally, with peak secretion at night for mammals, including humans. Melatonin is synthesized and released in response to norepinephrine, whose rate of release declines when light activates retinal photoreceptors. Melatonin release is decreased in women with *estrogen-receptor-positive* breast cancer. The significance of this reduced nocturnal release of melatonin is not well understood at this time.

MICROMETASTASIS. The occult spread of cancer cells to remote regions of the body apart from the site of original tumor.

MITOGEN. A substance that induces cell division and transformation, especially lymphocyte transformation.

NATURAL KILLER CELLS. Large granular lymphcytes that are cytotoxic without prior sensitization. Natural killer cells have a toxic effect on tumor cells as well as other target cells.

NEOPLASIA. Literally "new growth," a term commonly used to refer to cancer.

NEUROPEPTIDE. Molecules composed of short chains of amino acids found in both central nervous system and peripheral tissue (*enkephalins*, endorphines, vasopressins, and so on). Neuropeptides function as hormones but are also frequently classifed as neurotransmittors.

ONCOGENE. Viral genetic material carrying the potential for causing cancer when inappropriately activated.

OPIOIDS. Naturally occurring peptides (for example, the *enkephalins* or endorphines) that have opiate-like effects by binding to opiate receptors on cell membranes.

PENTOSAN (pentose fiber). A groups of pentose polysaccharides found in various plant juices and foods. Upon hydrolysis they yield pentose.

PHARMACOLOGICAL DOSE. Dose of drug achieving a physical effect beyond endogenous or normal limits of biochemicals within the organism.

PHOTOCARCINOGENESIS. Process by which cancer arises from exposure to ultraviolet radiation.

PHYSIOLOGICAL DOSE. Dose of drug that conforms to or mimics level of normal chemical functioning within the organism.

RECEPTOR. A specific molecule on the surface or within the cytoplasm of the cell that recognizes and binds with other specific molecules—for example, the molecules on the surface of an *immunocompetent cell* that bind with *antigen*.

RETROVIRUS. An infective agent that has RNA as its genetic material. In infected cells the RNA is copied into DNA, which may then become integrated into the genome of the host cell.

SARCOMA. A cancer arising from connective tissue. Sarcomas, such as osteosarcoma (cancer of the bone), are often highly malignant and epidemiologically have not been shown to be age linked.

SIGMOIDOSCOPY. Examination of the sigmoid region of the large bowel by means of a sigmoidoscope.

SQUAMOUS CELL CARCINOMA. A slightly elevated lesion, often with an irregular border and usually with chronic ulceration. Advanced lesions show large ulcerations, exhibiting scabs that do not heal.

SYNGENEIC. Having identical genetic typing—for example, tissues from animals of the same inbred strain or tissues from identical twins.

T CELLS (T lymphocytes). Thymus-derived, *immunocompetent cells* that participate in *cell-mediated immune reactions*.

T-HELPER CELLS. Effector T cells that cooperate with *B cells* in *antibody* formation. T-helper cells are functionally important for IgG, IgA, and IgE immune responses (see *immunoglobulins*).

T-SUPPRESSOR CELLS. Cells that specifically inhibit *antibody* production, as well as other cellular immune reactions by effector T cells. These cells are stimulated antigenically and are *antigen* specific in their suppression.

TITER. The quantity of a substance required to produce a reaction with a given volume of another substance, or the amount of one substance required to correspond with a given amount of another substance.

TUMOR GRADE. The grade of the tumor given by a pathologist, reflecting the degree of cellular differentiation of the cancer cell. Grades generally express the degree of cellular malignancy, and such pathology grading has been developed for a variety of tumors, including breast and bladder cancer, as well as *sarcomas*. Generally, the higher the grade, the more malignant or aggressive the tumor and hence the worst prognosis.

URINARY RIBOFLAVIN OUTPUT. A common measure of amount of fiber intake. Riboflavin, one of the B vitamins, is found in milk, muscle, liver, kidney, eggs, grass, malt, leafy young vegetables, and various algae and is an essential nutrient for man. Excreted riboflavin in the urine is discussed in the text as a measure of dietary fiber intake for participants in cancer prevention clinical trials.

References

Ader, R. (ed.). *Psychoneuroimmunology*. Orlando, Fla.: Academic Press, 1981.

Ader, R., and Friedman, S. B. "Differential Early Experiences and Susceptibility to Transplanted Tumor in the Rat." *Journal of Comparative and Physiological Psychology*, 1965, *59*, 361–364.

Ado, A., and Goldstein, M. M. "The Primary Immune Response in Rabbits After Lesion of the Different Zones in the Medial Hypothalamus." *Annals of Allergy*, 1973, *31*, 585–589.

Allegra, J., and others. "Association Between Steroid Hormone Receptor Status and Disease-Free Interval in Breast Cancer." *Cancer Treatment Reports*, 1979, *63*, 1271–1277.

Allison, S., and Wong, K. "Skin Cancer: Some Ethnic Differences." In J. Bresler (ed.), *Environments of Men*. Reading, Mass.: Addison-Wesley, 1967.

Alpert, L. C., Brawer, J. R., Patel, Y. C., and Reichlin, S. "Somatostatinergic Neurons in Anterior Hypothalamus: Immunohistochemical Localization." *Endocrinology*, 1976, *98*, 255–258.

American Cancer Society. *A Survey Concerning Cigarette Smoking, Health Check-Ups, Cancer Detection Tests: A Summary of the Findings*. DHEW Publication No. 79–1549. Bethesda, Md.: National Institutes of Health, 1979.

American Cancer Society. *Cancer Facts and Figures*. New York: American Cancer Society, 1981.

American Cancer Society. *Cancer Facts and Figures*. New York: American Cancer Society, 1985.

Ames, B. "Dietary Carcinogens and Anticarcinogens." *Science*, 1983, *221*, 1256–1264.

Anisman, H., and Lapierre, Y. "Neurochemical Aspects of Stress and Depression: Formulations and Caveats." In W. Neufeld (ed.), *Stress and Psychopathology*. New York: McGraw-Hill, 1980.

Antonovsky, A., and Hartman, H. "Delay in the Detection of Cancer: A Review of the Literature." *Health Education Monographs*, 1974, *2*, 98–128.

Aurelian, L., Strandberg, J., and Marcus, R. "Neutralization, Immuno-Fluorescence and Complement Fixation Tests in Identification of Antibody to Herpes Virus Type 2–Induced Tumor-Specific Antigen in Sera and Squamous Cervical Carcinoma." *Immunology and Cancer: Progress in Experimental Tumor Research*, 1974, *19*, 165–181.

Austin, D., and Roe, K. "Increase in Cancer of the Corpus Uteri in the San Francisco–Oakland Standard Metropolitan Statistical Area, 1960–1975." *Journal of the National Cancer Institute*, 1979, *62*, 13–16.

Aylsworth, C., Hodson, C., and Meites, J. "Opiate Antagonists Can Inhibit Mammary Tumor Growth in Rats." *Proceedings of the Society for Experimental Biology and Medicine*, 1979, *161*, 18–20.

Bach, F. H., and Hirschhorn, K. "The *in vitro* Immune Response of Peripheral Blood Lymphocytes." *Seminars in Hematology*, 1965, *2*, 68–89.

Baron, B., and Richart, R. "An Epidemiologic Study of Cervical Neoplastic Disease Based on a Self-Selected Sample of 7,000 Women in Barbados, West Indies." *Cancer*, 1971, *27*, 978–986.

Barré-Sinoussi, F., and others. "Isolation of a T-Lymphotropic Retrovirus from a Patient at Risk for Acquired Immune Deficiency Syndrome (AIDS)." *Science*, 1983, *220*, 868–871.

Bartrop, R.W., and others. "Depressed Lymphocyte Function After Bereavement." *Lancet*, 1977, *1*, 834–836.

Beatson, G. T. "On the Treatment of Inoperable Cases of Carcinoma of the Mammary: Suggestions for a New Method of Treatment with Illustrative Cases." *Lancet*, 1896, *2*, 104–107.

Becker, M., and Maiman, L. "Strategies for Enhancing Patient Compliance." *Journal of Community Health*, 1980, *6*, 113–135.

Bennett, R., and Robins, P. "On the Selection of a Sunscreen." *Journal of Dermatology and Surgical Oncology*, 1977, *3*, 205–209.

Beral, V. "Cancer of the Cervix: A Sexually Transmitted Infection?" *Lancet*, 1974, *1*, 1037–1040.

Berg, J., and Lampe, J. "High-Risk Factors in Gynecologic Cancer." *Cancer*, 1981, *48*, 429–441.

Berg, J., Ross, R., and Latourette, H. "Economic Status and Survival of Cancer Patients." *Cancer*, 1977, *39*, 467–477.

Berger, P., and Luckman, T. *The Social Construction of Reality*. New York: Doubleday, 1966.

Berkman, L., and Syme, L. "Social Networks, Host Resistance, and Mortality: A Nine-Year Follow-Up Study of Alameda County Residents." *American Journal of Epidemiology*, 1979, *2*, 186–204.

Bernstein, I., and Treneer, C. "Learned Food Aversions and Tumor Anorexia." In T. Burish, S. Levy, and B. Meyerwitz (eds.), *Cancer, Nutrition, and Eating Behavior*. Hillsdale, N.J.: Erlbaum, 1985.

Besedovsky, H., and Sorkin, E. "Network of Immunoneuroendocrine Interactions." *Clinical and Experimental Immunology*, 1977, *27*, 1–12.

Besedovsky, H., and others. "The Immune Response Evokes Changes in Brain Noradrenergic Neurons." *Science*, 1983, *221*, 564–566.

Bingham, S., Williams, D., Cole, T., and James, W. "Dietary Fibre and Regional Large-Bowel Cancer Mortality in Britain." *British Journal of Cancer*, 1979, *40*, 456–463.

Blalock, J. "The Immune System as a Sensory Organ." *Journal of Immunology*, 1984, *132*, 1067–1070.

Blecha, F., Kelley, K., and Satterlee, D. "Adrenal Involvement in the Expression of Delayed-Type Hypersensitivity to SRBC and Contact Sensitivity to DNFB in Stressed Mice." *Proceedings of the Society for Experimental Biology and Medicine*, 1982, *169*, 247–252.

Blum, H. "Ultraviolet Radiation and Skin Cancer in Mice and Men: Accumulation of Effect and Uncertainty of Prediction." *National Cancer Institute Monograph*, 1978, *50*, 11–12.

Bonadonna, G., and Valagussa, P. "Dose-Response Affect of Adjuvant Chemotherapy in Breast Cancer." *New England Journal of Medicine*, 1981, *304*, 10–15.

Borthwick, N. M., and Bell, P. A. (eds.). *Glucocorticoid Action and Leukemia*. Cardiff: Alpha Omega Alpha Publishing, 1978.

Bosl, G., and others. "Impact of Delay in Diagnosis on Clinical Stage of Testicular Cancer." *Lancet*, 1981, *2*, 970–973.

Bourne, H. R., Lichtenstein, L. M., and Melmon, K. L. "Modulation of Inflammation and Immunity by Cyclic AMP." *Science*, 1974, *184*, 9–28.

Boyd, N. "Pilot Study of Dietary Fat Reduction in High Risk Women." In T. Burish, S. Levy, and B. Meyerwitz (eds.), *Cancer, Nutrition, and Eating Behavior: A Biobehavioral Perspective*. Hillsdale, N.J.: Erlbaum, 1985.

Braun, A. *The Story of Cancer*. Reading, Mass.: Addison-Wesley, 1977.

Bright-See, E., and Levy, S. "Dietary Intervention in Cancer Prevention Trials and Clinical Practice: Some Methodological Issues." In T. Burish, S. Levy, and B. Meyerwitz (eds.), *Cancer, Nutrition, and Eating Behavior: A Biobehavioral Perspective*. Hillsdale, N.J.: Erlbaum, 1985.

Brooks, W. H., Netsky, M. G., Normansell, D. E., and Horwitz, D. A. "Depressed Cell Mediated Immunity in Patients with Primary Intracranial Tumors." *Journal of Experimental Medicine*, 1972, *136*, 1631–1647.

Brown, G. M., and Reichlin, S. "Psychologic and Neural Regulation of Growth Hormone Secretion." *Psychosomatic Medicine*, 1972, *34*, 45–61.

Brownstein, M. "Minireview: The Pineal Gland." *Life Sciences*, 1975, *16*, 1363–1374.

Buckley, J., Harris, R., Doll, R., and Williams, P. "Case-Control Study of the Husbands of Women with Dysplasia or Carcinoma of the Cervix Uteri." *Lancet*, 1981, *2*, 1010–1015.

Bulloch, K., and Moore, R. Y. "Nucleus Ambiguous Projections to the Thymus Gland—Possible Pathways for Regulation of the Immune Response and the Neuroendocrine Network." *Abstracts of the American Association of Anatomy*, 1980, 25A.

Burish, T., Levy, S., and Meyerwitz, B. (eds.). *Cancer, Nutrition, and Eating Behavior: A Biobehavioral Perspective*. Hillsdale, N.J.: Erlbaum, 1985.

Burns, B. "Chronic Chest Disease, Personality and Success in Stopping Cigarette Smoking." *British Journal of Preventive Social Medicine*, 1969, *23*, 23–27.

Calabrese, E. "Is the Role of the Environment in Carcinogenesis Overestimated?" *Medical Hypotheses*, 1979, *5*, 5–14.

Calvo, W. "The Innervation of the Bone Marrow in Laboratory Animals." *American Journal of Anatomy*, 1968, *123*, 315–328.

Carney, D. N., and others. "Selective Growth in Serum-Free Hormone-Supplemented Medium of Tumor Cells Obtained by Biopsy from Patients with Small Cell Carcinoma of the Lung." *Proceedings of the National Academy of Sciences*, 1981, *78*, 3185–3190.

Carroll, B. J., and others. "A Specific Laboratory Test for the Diagnosis of Melancholia." *Archives of General Psychiatry*, 1981, *34*, 15–22.

Cassileth, B. "After Laetrile, What?" *New England Journal of Medicine*, 1982, *306*, 1482–1484.

Cassileth, B., Zupkis, R., Sutton-Smith, K., and March, V. "Informed Consent: Why Are Its Goals Imperfectly Realized?" *New England Journal of Medicine*, 1980, *302*, 896–900.

Catalano, L., and Johnson, L. "Herpes Virus Antibody and Carcinoma *in situ* of the Cervix." *Journal of the American Medical Association*, 1971, *217*, 447–450.

Celentano, D., Shapiro, S., and Weisman, C. "Cancer Preventive Screening of Behavior Among Elderly Women." *Preventive Medicine*, 1982, *11*, 454–463.

Chrombie, I. "Variation of Melanoma Incidence with Latitude in North America and Europe." *British Journal of Cancer*, 1979, *40*, 774–781.

Claman, H. N. "Corticosteroids and Lymphoid Cells." *New England Journal of Medicine*, 1972, *287*, 388–397.

Clayton, P. J. "The Sequelae and Nonsequelae of Conjugal

Bereavement." *American Journal of Psychiatry*, 1979, *136*, 1530–1534.

Cleaver, J. "Xeroderma Pigmentosum: Genetic and Environmental Influences in Skin Carcinogenesis." *International Journal of Dermatology*, 1978, *17*, 435–449.

Cochran, A. *Man, Cancer, and Immunity*. Orlando, Fla.: Academic Press, 1978.

Coe, C., and Levine, S. "Normal Responses to Mother-Infant Separation in Nonhuman Primates." In D. Klein and J. Rabkin (eds.), *Anxiety: New Research and Changing Concepts*. New York: Raven Press, 1981.

Coe, C., Wiener, S., and Levine, S. "Normal Responses of Mother and Infant Monkeys to Disturbance and Separation." In H. Moltz and L. Rosenblum (eds.), *Symbiosis in Parent-Young Interactions*. New York: Plenum, 1983.

Coe, C., Wiener, S., Rosenberg, L., and Levine, S. "Endocrine and Immune Responses to Separation and Maternal Loss in Non-Human Primates." In M. Reite and T. Fields (eds.), *Psychology of Attachment*. Orlando, Fla.: Academic Press, 1985.

Cohen, M., Chabner, B., and Lippman, M. "Role of Pineal Gland in Aetiology and Treatment of Breast Cancer." *Lancet*, 1978, *2*, 814–816.

Cohen, J., and Cohen, P. *Applied Multiple Regression/Correlation Analysis for the Behavioral Sciences*. New York: Wiley, 1975.

Cole, P. "Cancer and Occupation: Status and Needs of Epidemiologic Research." *Cancer*, 1977, *39*, 1788–1791.

Cole, P., and Austin, H. "Breast Self-Examination: An Adjuvant to Early Cancer Detection." *American Journal of Public Health*, 1981, *71*, 572–578.

Committee on Diet, Nutrition, and Cancer, National Academy of Sciences. *Diet, Nutrition, and Cancer*. Washington, D. C.: National Academy Press, 1982.

Connor, W., Connor, S., Fry, M., and Warner, S. *The Alternative Diet Book*. Iowa City: University of Iowa Press, 1980.

Cooper, H., Patchefsky, A., and Marks, G. "Cloacogenic Carcinoma of the Anorectum in Homosexual Men: An Observation of Four Cases." *Diseases of the Colon and Rectum*, 1979, *22*, 557–558.

Copeland, E., and Dudrick, S. "Nutritional Aspects of Cancer." In C. Hickey (ed.), *Current Problems in Cancer.* Vol. 1. Chicago: Year Book Medical Publishers, 1976.

Costa, G., and Donaldson, S. "The Nutritional Effects of Cancer and Its Therapy." *Nutrition and Cancer*, 1980, *2*, 22-29.

Cowie, B. "The Cardiac Patient's Perception of His Heart Attack." *Social Sciences and Medicine*, 1976, *10*, 87-96.

Cox, B. "Endogenous Opioid Peptides: A Guide to Structure and Terminology." *Life Sciences*, 1982, *31*, 1645-1658.

Cox, T., and MacKay, C. "Psychosocial Factors and Psychophysiological Mechanisms in the Etiology and Development of Cancers." *Social Science and Medicine*, 1982, *16*, 381-396.

Criep, L. H. *Clinical Immunology and Allergy.* Orlando, Fla.: Grune & Stratton, 1969.

Cross, R. J., Markesbery, W. R., Brooks, W. H., and Roszman, T. L. "Hypothalamic-Immune Interactions: The Acute Effect of Anterior Hypothalamic Lesions on the Immune Response." *Brain Research*, 1980, *196*, 79-87.

Cummings, K., Becker, M., Kirscht, J., and Levin, N. "Intervention Strategies to Improve Compliance with Medical Regimes by Ambulatory Hemodialysis Patients." *Journal of Behavioral Medicine*, 1981, *4*, 111-127.

Danforth, D., Tamarkin, L., Do, R., and Lippman, M. "Melatonin-Induced Increase in Cytoplasmic Estrogen Receptor Activity in Hamster Uteri." *Endocrinology*, 1983, *113*, 81-85.

Denckla, W. D. "Interactions Between Age and Neuroendocrine and Immune Systems." *Federation Proceedings*, 1978, *37*, 1263-1266.

del Rey, A., Besedovsky, H., and Sorkin, E. "Endogenous Blood Levels of Corticosterone Control the Immunologic Cell Mass and B Cell Activity in Mice." *Journal of Immunology*, 1984, *133*, 572-575.

Dennis, C., Gardner, B., and Lim, B. "Analysis of Survival and Recurrence vs. Patient and Doctor Delay in Treatment of Breast Cancer." *Cancer*, 1975, *35*, 714-720.

Dent, O., Bartrop, R., Goulston, K., and Chapuis, P. "Participating in Faecal Occult Blood Screening for Colorectal Cancer." *Social Sciences and Medicine*, 1983, *17*, 17–23.

Derogatis, L. R., Abeloff, M. D., and Melisaratos, N. "Psychological Coping Mechanisms and Survival Time in Metastatic Breast Cancer." *Journal of the American Medical Association*, 1979, *242*, 1504–1509.

DeWys, W. "Pathophysiology of Cancer Cachexia: Current Understanding and Areas for Future Research." *Cancer Research*, 1982, *42* (supp.), 721S–726S.

DiClemente, R., and others. "Patient Delay in the Diagnosis of Cancer Emphasizing Malignant Melanoma of the Skin." In C. Mettlin and G. Murphy (eds.), *Issues in Cancer Screening and Communications*. New York: Alan R. Liss, 1982.

Dilman, V. M. "Metabolic Immunodepression Which Increases the Risk of Cancer." *Lancet*, 1977, *2*, 1207–1209.

Dolan, T. "Cancer of the Female Genital Tract." In P. Rubin (ed.), *Clinical Oncology for Medical Students and Physicians*. New York: American Cancer Society, 1978.

Doll, R., and Peto, R. "Mortality in Relation to Smoking: 20 Years' Observations on Male British Doctors." *British Medical Journal*, 1976, *2*, 1525–1536.

Doll, R., and Peto, R. *The Causes of Cancer*. New York: Oxford University Press, 1981.

Donaldson, S. "Effects of Therapy on Nutritional Status of the Pediatric Cancer Patient." *Cancer Research*, 1982, *42*, 729–734.

Dunbar, Q., and Stunkard, A. "Adherence to Diet and Drug Regime." In R. Levy and others (eds.), *Nutrition, Lipids and Coronary Heart Disease*. New York: Raven Press, 1979.

Durnberger, H., and others. "Mesenchyme-Mediated Effect of Testosterone on Embryonic Mammary Epithelium." *Cancer Research*, 1978, *38*, 4066–4069.

Eddy, D., and Eddy, J. "Delay Factors in the Detection of Cancer." In *Proceedings of the Fourth National Conference on Human Values and Cancer*. New York: American Cancer Society, 1984.

Editorial. *Journal of the American Medical Association*, 1983, *249*, 2375–2376.

Eidinger, D., and Garrett, T. J. "Studies in the Regulatory Effects of the Sex Hormones on Antibody Formation and

Stem Cell Differentiation." *Journal of Experimental Medicine*, 1972, *136*, 1098–1116.

Elwood, J., and Moorehead, W. "Delay in Diagnosis and Long-Term Survival in Breast Cancer." *British Medical Journal*, 1980, *280*, 1291–1294.

Epstein, J. "Photocarcinogenesis: A Review." *National Cancer Institute Monograph*, 1978, *50*, 13–25.

Epstein, L., and Cluss, P. "A Behavioral Medicine Perspective on Adherence to Long-Term Medical Regimens." *Journal of Consulting and Clinical Psychology*, 1982, *50*, 950–971.

Epstein, S. *The Politics of Cancer*. New York: Doubleday, 1979.

Eskola, J., and others. "Effect of Sport Stress on Lymphocyte Transformation and Antibody Formation." *Clinical and Experimental Immunology*, 1978, *32*, 339–345.

Evans, R., and others. "Deterring the Onset of Smoking in Children: Knowledge of Immediate Physiological Effects and Coping with Peer Pressure, Media Pressure, and Parent Modeling." *Journal of Applied Social Psychology*, 1978, *8*, 126–135.

Everson, T., and Cole, W. *Spontaneous Aggression of Cancer*. Philadelphia: Saunders, 1966.

Fauci, A. S. "Corticosteroids and Circulating Lymphocytes." *Transplantation Proceedings*, 1975, *7*, 37–48.

Fauci, A. S., and Dale, D. C. "The Effect of Hydrocortisone on the Kinetics of Normal Human Lymphocytes." *Blood*, 1975, *46*, 235–243.

Feifel, H. *New Meanings of Death*. New York: McGraw-Hill, 1977.

Ferguson, R. M., Schmidtke, J. R., and Simmons, R. L. "Inhibition of Mitogen Induced Lymphocyte Transformation by Local Anesthetics." *Journal of Immunology*, 1976, *116*, 627–634.

Fessel, W. J. "Mental Stress, Blood Proteins, and the Hypothalamus." *Archives of General Psychiatry*, 1962, *7*, 427–435.

Filipp, G., and Mess, B. "Role of the Adrenocortical System in Suppressing Anaphylaxis After Hypothalamic Lesion." *Annals of Allergy*, 1969, *27*, 607–610.

Filipp, G., and Szentivanyi, A. "Anaphylaxis and the Nervous System: Part III." *Annals of Allergy*, 1958, *16*, 306–311.

Fisher, E., Redmond, C., and Fisher, B. "A Perspective Concerning the Relation of Duration of Symptoms to Treatment Failure in Patients with Breast Cancer." *Cancer*, 1977, *40*, 3160-3167.

Fletcher, J., Branson, R., and Freireich, E. "Ethical Considerations in Clinical Trials: Invited Remarks." *Clinical Pharmacology and Therapeutics*, 1979, *25*, 742-746.

Folkman, J., and Haudenschild, C. "Angiogenesis *in vitro*." *Nature*, 1980, *288*, 551-555.

Forbes, P. "Photocarcinogenesis: An Overview." *Journal of Investigative Dermatology*, 1981, *77*, 139-143.

Forbes, P., Davies, R., and Urbach, F. "Aging, Environmental Influences, and Photocarcinogenesis." *Journal of Investigative Dermatology*, 1979, *73*, 131-134.

Fox, B. "Premorbid Psychological Factors as Related to Cancer Incidence." *Journal of Behavioral Medicine*, 1978, *1*, 45-133.

Fox, B. "Behavioral Issues in Cancer." In S. Weiss, J. Herd, and B. Fox (eds.), *Perspectives on Behavioral Medicine*. Orlando, Fla.: Academic Press, 1981.

Frankenhaeuser, M. "Experimental Approaches to the Study of Human Behavior as Related to Neuroendocrine Functions." In L. Levi (ed.), *Society, Stress, and Disease*. Vol. 1. New York: Oxford University Press, 1971.

Freedman, D. X., and Fenichel, G. "Effect of Midbrain Lesion on Experimental Allergy." *Archives of Neurological Psychiatry*, 1958, *79*, 164-169.

Freeman, H. "Success of Differential Disease Outcome in Population Subgroups: Changing the Odds in the Inner City." Paper presented at workshop on Behavioral Aspects of Screening and Early Detection of Cancer, Bethesda, Md., Aug. 26-27, 1982.

Friedman, G., Petiti, D., Bawol, R., and Siegelaub, A. "Mortality in Cigarette Smokers and Quitters." *New England Journal of Medicine*, 1981, *364*, 1407-1410.

Frohman, L. A. "Ectopic Hormone Production." *American Journal of Medicine*, 1981, *70*, 995-999.

Frost, P., and Kerbel, R. "Immunology of Metastasis: Can the Immune Response Cope with Disseminated Tumor?" *Cancer Metastasis Reviews*, 1983, *2*, 239-256.

Funch, D., and Marshall, J. "The Role of Stress, Social Support and Age in Survival from Breast Cancer." *Journal of Psychosomatic Research*, 1983, *27*, 177–183.

Funch, D., and Mettlin, C. "The Role of Support in Relation to Recovery from Breast Surgery." *Social Science and Medicine*, 1982, *16*, 91–98.

Gallo, R., and others. "Frequent Detection and Isolation of Cytopathic Retroviruses (HTLV-III) from Patients with AIDS and at Risk for AIDS." *Science*, 1984, *224*, 500–503.

Gardner, J., and Lyon, J. "Cancer in Utah Mormon Men by Lay Priesthood Level." *American Journal of Epidemiology*, 1982a, *116*, 243–257.

Gardner, J., and Lyon, J. "Cancer in Utah Mormon Women by Church Activity Level." *American Journal of Epidemiology*, 1982b, *116*, 258–265.

Garfield, C. (ed.). *Psychosocial Care of the Dying Patient*. Hawthorne, N.Y.: Aldine, 1978.

Garfinkel, L. "Cancer Mortality in Nonsmokers: Prospective Study by the American Cancer Society." *Journal of the National Cancer Institute*, 1980, *65*, 1169–1173.

Garfinkel, L. "Time Trends in Lung Cancer Mortality Among Nonsmokers and a Note on Passive Smoking." *Journal of the National Cancer Institute*, 1981, *66*, 1061–1066.

Giron, L. T., Crutcher, K. A., and Davis, J. N. "Lymph Nodes—A Possible Site for Sympathetic Neuronal Regulation of Immune Responses." *Annals of Neurology*, 1980, *8*, 520–555.

Gisler, R. H. "Stress and the Hormonal Regulation of the Immune Response in Mice." *Psychotherapy and Psychosomatics*, 1974, *23*, 197–208.

Gold, W. M. "Cholinergic Pharmacology in Asthma." In K. F. Austen and L. M. Lichtenstein (eds.), *Asthma Physiology, Immuno-Pharmacology and Treatment*. Orlando, Fla.: Academic Press, 1973.

Gordis, L., Markowitz, M., and Lillienfeld, A. "The Inaccuracy of Using Interviews to Estimate Patient Reliability in Taking Medication at Home." *Medical Care*, 1969, *7*, 49–54.

Gottlieb, M., and others. "*Pneumocystis Carinii* Pneumonia and

Mucosal Candidiasis in Previously Healthy Homosexual Men." *New England Journal of Medicine*, 1981, *305*, 1425–1431.

Gould-Martin, K., and others. "Behavioral and Biological Determinants of Surgical Stage of Breast Cancer." *Preventive Medicine*, 1982, *11*, 429–440.

Graham, S., Rawls, W., Swanson, M., and McCurtis, J. "Sex Partners and Herpes Simplex Virus Type 2 in the Epidemiology of Cancer of the Cervix." *American Journal of Epidemiology*, 1982, *115*, 729–735.

Gray, B. *Human Subjects in Medical Experimentation*. New York: Wiley, 1975.

Green, L., Levine, D., and Deeds, S. "Clinical Trials of Health Education for Hypertensive Outpatients: Design and Baseline Data." *Preventive Medicine*, 1975, *4*, 417–425.

Greenberg, A., Dyck, D., and Sandler, L. "Opponent Processes, Neurohormones and Natural Resistance." In B. Fox and B. Newberry (eds.), *Psychoneuroendocrine Systems in Cancer and Immunity*. Toronto: Hogrefe, 1984.

Greene, W. A. "The Psychosocial Setting of the Development of Leukemia and Lymphoma." *Annals of the New York Academy of Sciences*, 1966, *129*, 794–806.

Greenwald, H., Becker, S., and Nevitt, M. "Delay and Noncompliance in Cancer Detection." *Health and Society*, 1978, *56*, 212–230.

Greer, S., Morris, T., and Pettingale, K. "Psychological Response to Breast Cancer: Effect on Outcome." *Lancet*, 1979, *2*, 785–787.

Greer, S., Morris, T., Pettingale, K., and Haybittle, J. "Mental Attitudes to Cancer: An Additional Prognostic Factor." *Lancet*, 1985, *1*, 750.

Grundner, T. "On the Readability of Surgical Consent Forms." *New England Journal of Medicine*, 1980, *302*, 900–901.

Guinan, P., and others. "What Is the Best Test to Detect Prostate Cancer?" *Ca-A Cancer Journal for Clinicians*, 1981, *31*, 141–145.

Hackett, T., Cassem, N., and Raker, J. "Patient Delay in Cancer." *New England Journal of Medicine*, 1973, *289*, 1–54.

Hagnell, O. "The Premorbid Personality of Persons Who Develop Cancer in a Total Population Investigated in 1947 and 1957." *Annals of the New York Academy of Sciences*, 1966, *125*, 846–855.

Hammond, E., Garfinkel, L., and Seidman, H. "Some Recent Findings Concerning Cigarette Smoking." In H. Haite, J. Watson, and J. Winsten (eds.), *Origins of Human Cancer*. Cold Spring Harbor, N.Y.: Cold Spring Harbor Laboratory, 1977.

Handel, S. "Change in Smoking Habits in a General Practice." *Postgraduate Medicine*, 1973, *49*, 679–681.

Hanna, N., and Burton, R. "Definitive Evidence That Natural Killer (NK) Cells Inhibit Experimental Tumor Metastasis *in vivo*." *Journal of Immunology*, 1981, *127*, 1754–1758.

Hanna, N., and Fidler, I. "Role of Natural Killer Cells in the Destruction of Circulating Tumor Emboli." *Journal of the National Cancer Institute*, 1980, *65*, 801–809.

Haverkos, H., and Curran, J. "The Current Outbreak of Kaposi's Sarcoma and Opportunistic Infections." *Ca-A Cancer Journal for Clinicians*, 1982, *32*, 330–339.

Haynes, B., Taylor, D., and Sackett, D. *Compliance in Health Care*. Baltimore: Johns Hopkins University Press, 1979.

Hein, K., Schreiber, K., Cohen, M., and Koss, L. "Cervical Cytology: The Need for Routine Screening in the Sexually Active Adolescent." *Adolescent Medicine*, 1977, *91*, 123–126.

Henderson, C., and Canellos, G. "Cancer of the Breast: The Past Decade. Parts I and II." *New England Journal of Medicine*, 1980, *302*, 17–30, 78–90.

Henney, J. "Unproven Methods of Cancer Treatment." In V. DeVita, S. Hellman, and S. Rosenberg (eds.), *Principles and Practice of Oncology*. Philadelphia: Lippincott, 1982.

Henry, J. "The Relation of Social to Biological Processes in Disease." *Social Science and Medicine*, 1982, *16*, 369–380.

Herberman, R., and Ortaldo, J. "Natural Killer Cells: Their Role in Defenses Against Disease." *Science*, 1981, *214*, 24–30.

Herberman, R., and Santoni, A. "Regulation of Natural Killer Cell Activity." In E. Mihich (ed.), *Biological Responses in Cancer*. Vol 2. New York: Plenum, 1984.

Herd, A., Weiss, S., and Fox, B. (eds.). *Perspectives on Behavioral Medicine*. Orlando, Fla.: Academic Press, 1981.

Hill, C. W., Greer, W. E., and Felsenfeld, O. "Psychological Stress, Early Response to Foreign Protein, and Blood Cortisol in Vervets." *Psychosomatic Medicine*, 1967, *29*, 279–283.

Hirata-Hibi, M. "Plasma Cell Reaction and Thymic Germinal Centers After a Chronic Form of Electric Stress." *Journal of the Reticuloendothelioma Society*, 1967, *4*, 370–389.

Hirayama, T. "Non-Smoking Wives of Heavy Smokers Have a Higher Risk of Lung Cancer: A Study from Japan." *British Medical Journal*, 1981, *282*, 183–185.

Hoagland, A., Morrow, G., Bennett, J., and Carnrike, C. "Oncologists' Views of Cancer Patient Noncompliance." *American Journal of Clinical Oncology*, 1983, *6*, 239–244.

Holmes, T. H., and Masuda, M. "Life Changes and Illness Susceptibility." In B. S. Dohrenwend and B. P. Dohrenwend (eds.), *Stressful Life Events: Their Nature and Effects*. New York; Wiley, 1974.

Holtzman, D., and Celentano, D. "The Practice and Efficacy of Breast Self-Examination: A Critical Review." *American Journal of Public Health*, 1983, *73*, 1324–1326.

Howard, J. "In-Reach: An Approach to the Secondary Prevention of Cancer." In *Behavior, Health Risks, and Social Disadvantage*. Washington, D.C.: National Academy Press, 1982a.

Howard, J. "Breast Self-Examination: Issues for Research." Proceedings of the Working Group Meeting to Explore Issues in Breast Self-Examination. Bethesda, Md., Apr. 19–20, 1982b.

Huggins, C., and Hodges, C. V. "Studies in Prostate Cancer: The Effect of Castration, of Estrogen and Androgen Injection on Serum Phosphatases in Metastatic Carcinoma of the Prostate." *Cancer Research*, 1941, *1*, 293–297.

Hulka, B. "Risk Factors for Cervical Cancer." *Journal of Chronic Diseases*, 1982, *35*, 3–11.

Humphrey, L., Singla, O., and Volence, F. "Immunologic Responsiveness of the Breast Cancer Patient." *Cancer*, 1980, *46*, 893–898.

Ikeda, T., and Sirbasku, D. A. "Purification and Properties of a Mammary-Uterine Pituitary Tumor Cell Growth Factor from Pregnant Sheep Uterus." *Biological Chemistry*, 1984, *259*, 4049-4064.

Jankovic, B. D., Jovanova, K., and Markovic, B. M. "Effect of Hypothalamic Stimulation on the Immune Reactions in the Rat." *Periodicum Biologorum*, 1979, *81*, 211-212.

Jemmott, J., and Locke, S. "Psychosocial Factors, Immunologic Mediation, and Human Susceptibility to Infectious Diseases: How Much Do We Know?" *Psychological Bulletin*, 1984, *95*, 78-108.

Jensen, M. "Psychobiological Factors in the Prognosis and Treatment of Neoplastic Disorders." Unpublished doctoral dissertation, Department of Psychology, Yale University, 1984.

Jick, H., Walter, A., and Rothman, K. "The Epidemic of Endometrial Cancer: A Commentary." *American Journal of Public Health*, 1980, *70*, 264-267.

Joasoo, A., and McKenzie, J. M. "Stress and the Immune Response in Rats." *International Archives of Allergy and Applied Immunology*, 1976, *50*, 659-663.

Johnson, P., Armor, D., Polich, S., and Stambul, H. *U.S. Adult Drinking Practices: Time Trends, Social Correlates and Sex Roles*. Santa Monica, Calif.: Rand, 1977.

Kahn, H. "The DOM Study of Smoking and Mortality Among U.S. Veterans: Report on Eight and One-Half Years of Observation." *National Cancer Institute Monograph*, 1966, *19*, 1-125.

Kakidani, H., and others. "Cloning and Sequence Analysis of cDNA for Procine B-Neo-Endorphin/Dymorphin Precursor." *Nature*, 1982, *298*, 245-249.

Kappas, A., Jones, H. E. H., and Roitt, I. M. "Effects of Steroid Sex Hormones on Immunological Phenomena." *Nature*, 1963, *198*, 902.

Kastenbaum, R. "'Healthy Dying': A Paradoxical Quest Continues." *Journal of Social Issues*, 1979, *35*, 185-207.

Kegeles, S., and Grady, K. "Behavioral Dimensions." In D. Schottenfeld and J. Fraumeni (eds.), *Cancer Epidemiology and Prevention*. Philadelphia: Saunders, 1982.

Keller, S. E., and others. "Suppression of Lymphocyte Stimulation by Anterior Hypothalamic Lesions in the Guinea Pig." *Cellular Immunology*, 1980, *52*, 334-340.

Keller, S. E., and others. "Effect of Premature Weaning on Lymphocyte Stimulation in the Rat." *Psychosomatic Medicine*, 1983a, *45*, 75.

Keller, S. E., and others. "Stress-Induced Suppression of Immunity in Adrenalectomized Rats." *Science*, 1983b, *221*, 1301–1304.

Kelsey, J. L., and others. "Oral Contraceptives and Breast Disease: An Epidemiological Study." *Epidemiology*, 1978, *107*, 236–244.

Khansari, N., Whitten, N., and Fudenberg, N. "Phencyclidine-Induced Immunodepression." *Science*, 1984, *225*, 76–78.

Kikuchi, K., Ishii, Y., Veno, H., and Koshiba, H. "Cell-Mediated Immunity Involved in Autochthonous Tumor Rejection in Rats." *Annals of the New York Academy of Sciences*, 1976, *276*, 188–206.

Kimzey, S. L., Johnson, P. C., Ritzman, S. E., and Mengel, C. E. "Hematology and Immunology Studies: The Second Manned Skylab Mission." *Aviation and Space Environment Medicine*, 1976, *47*, 383–390.

Kittas, C., and Henry, L. "Effect of Sex Hormones on the Immune System of Guinea-Pigs and on the Development of Toxoplasmic Lesions in Non-Lymphoid Organs." *Clinical and Experimental Immunology*, 1979, *36*, 16–23.

Knopf, A. "Changes in Women's Opinions About Cancer." *Social Issues and Medicine*, 1976, *10*, 191–195.

Kobasa, S., Maddi, S., and Kahn, S. "Hardiness and Health: A Prospective Study." *Journal of Personality and Social Psychology*, 1982, *42*, 168–177.

Koller, E. A. "Atmung und Kreislauf in anaphylaktisch Enasthma Bronchiale des Meerschweinchens. III: Die Lunge Veränderungen in Asthmaanfall und die inspiratorische Reaction" [Respiration and Circulation in Anaphylactic Enasthma of the Bronchial Tubes of the Guinea Pig. III: The Lungs During an Asthma Attack and the Repiratory Response]. *Helvetica Physiologica Pharmacologica Acta*, 1968, *26*, 153–170.

Koop, C., and Luoto, J. " 'The Health Consequences of Smoking: Cancer.' Overview of Report of the Surgeon General." *Public Health Reports*, 1982, *97*, 318–324.

Korneva, E. A., and Khai, L. M. "Effect of Destruction of

Hypothalamic Areas on Immunogenesis." *Federation Proceedings* (supp.), 1964, *23*, 88–92.

Krakowski, A., Tur, E., and Brenner, S. "Multiple Agminated Juvenile Melanoma: A Case with a Sunburn History, and a Review." *Dermatologica*, 1981, *163*, 270–275.

Kress, D. *The Cigarette as a Physician Sees It*. Mountain View, Calif.: Pauper Press, 1931.

Kripke, M., and Fisher, M. "Immunologic Parameters of Ultraviolet Carcinogenesis." *Journal of the National Cancer Institute*, 1976, *57*, 211–215.

Kripke, M., and Fisher, M. "Immunologic Aspects of Tumor Induction by Ultraviolet Radiation." *National Cancer Institute Monograph*, 1978, *50*, 179–183.

Kronfol, Z., Silva, J., Jr., and Greden, J. "Impaired Lymphocyte Function in Depressive Illness." *Life Sciences*, 1983, *33*, 241–247.

Kübler-Ross, E. *On Death and Dying*. New York: Macmillan, 1969.

Kumakiri, A., Hashimoto, K., and Willis, I. "Biological Changes Due to a Long-Wave Ultraviolet Irradiation on Human Skin: Ultrastructure Study." *Journal of Investigative Dermatology*, 1977, *69*, 392–400.

Lancaster, H. "Some Geographical Aspects of the Mortality from Melanoma in Europeans." *Medical Journal of Australia*, 1956, *1*, 1082–1087.

Laudenslager, M., and Reite, M. "Coping and Separations: Immunological Consequences and Health Implications." In P. Sharer (ed.), *Review of Personality and Social Psychology*. Vol. 5: *Special Issue on Emotions, Relationships, and Health*. Beverly Hills, Calif.: Sage, 1984.

Laudenslager, M. L., and others. "Coping and Immunosuppression: Inescapable but Not Escapable Shock Suppresses Lymphocyte Proliferation." *Science*, 1983, *221*, 568–570.

Lazlo, J., Lucas, V., and Huang, A. "Iatrogenic Emesis Model in Cancer: Results of 120 Patients Treated with Delta-9-Tetrahydrocannabinol." In D. Foster (ed.), *The Treatment of Nausea and Vomiting Induced by Cancer Chemotherapy*. New York: Masson, 1981.

Lee, J., Marks, J., and Simpson, J. "Recruitment of Patients to Cooperative Group Clinical Trials." *Cancer Clinical Trials*, 1980, *3*, 381–384.

Leger, J., and Masson, G. "Factors Influencing an Anaphylactoid Reaction in the Rat." *Federation Proceedings*, 1947, *6*, 150–151.

LeShan, L. "Psychological States as Factors in the Development of Malignant Disease: A Critical Review." *Journal of the National Cancer Institute*, 1959, *22*, 1–18.

Leventhal, H., and Cleary, P. "The Smoking Problem: A Review of the Research and Theory in Behavioral Risk Modification." *Psychological Bulletin*, 1980, *88*, 370–405.

Levine, A., and others. "Controlled Clinical Trials of Nutritional Intervention as an Adjunct to Chemotherapy, with a Comment on Nutrition and Drug Resistance." *Cancer Research* (supp.), 1982, *42*, 774S–778S.

Levine, S., and Cohen, C. "Differential Survival to Leukemia as a Function of Infantile Stimulation in DB A/Z Mice." *Proceedings of the Society for Experimental Biology and Medicine*, 1959, *102*, 53–54.

Levy, J., and others. "Isolation of Lymphocytopathic Retroviruses from San Francisco Patients with AIDS." *Science*, 1984, *225*, 840–842.

Levy, S. "The Experience of Undergoing a Heart Attack: The Construction of a New Reality." *Journal of Phenomenological Psychology*, 1981, *12*, 153–171.

Levy, S. (ed.). *Biological Mediators of Behavior and Disease: Neoplasia.* New York: Elsevier Science, 1982.

Levy, S., and Howard, J., "Pattern T-Center Technologies: A Clinical-Cultural Perspective." In T. Miller, C. Green, and R. Meagher (eds.), *Handbook of Clinical Health Psychology.* New York: Plenum, 1982.

Levy, S., and others. "Prognostic Risk Assessment in Primary Breast Cancer by Behavioral and Immunological Parameters." *Health Psychology*, 1985, *4*, 99–113.

Lew, E., and Garfinkel, L. "Variations in Mortality by Weight Among 750,000 Men and Women." *Journal of Chronic Diseases*, 1979, *32*, 563–576.

Lewis, C., Linet, M., and Abeloff, M. "Compliance with Cancer Therapy by Patients and Physicians." *The American Journal of Medicine*, 1983, *74*, 673-678.

Lewis, C., and Michnich, M. "Contracts as a Means of Improving Patient Compliance." In I. Barofsky (ed.), *Medication Compliance: A Behavioral Management Approach*. Thorofare, N.J.: Slack, 1977.

Lewison, E. "Spontaneous Regression of Breast Cancer." *National Cancer Institute Monograph*, 1976, *44*, 23-25.

Lichtenstein, E., and Danaher, B. "Modification of Smoking Behavior: A Critical Analysis of Theory, Research, and Practice." In M. Hersen, R. Eisler, and P. Miller (eds.), *Progress in Behavior Modification*. Vol. 3. Orlando, Fla.: Academic Press, 1976.

Lidz, C., and others. *Informed Consent*. New York: Guilford Press, 1984.

Lieberman, S. *A Basic Study of Public Attitudes Toward Cancer and Cancer Tests*. Vol. 1: *Major Results*. New York: Lieberman Research, Inc., 1979.

Lilleyman, J., French, A., and Young, I. "Variation in 17 Oxogenic Steriod Excretion Following Oral Prednisolone in Children with Lymphoblastic Leukemia." *Oncology*, 1981, *38*, 274-276.

Lippman, M. E. "Hormonal Regulation of Human Breast Cancer Cells *in vitro*." In M. C. Pike, P. Siiteri, and C. W. Welsch (eds.), *Hormones and Breast Cancer*. Cold Spring Harbor, N.Y.: Cold Spring Harbor Laboratory, 1981.

Lippman, M. E. "Endocrine Responsive Cancers in Man." In R. Williams (ed.), *Textbook of Endocrinology*. Philadelphia: Saunders, 1985.

Lippman, M. E., Strobl, J., and Allegra, J. C. "Effects of Hormones on Human Breast Cancer Cells in Tissue Culture." In C. McGrath, M. Brennan, and M. Rich (eds.), *Cell Biology of Breast Cancer*. Orlando, Fla.: Academic Press, 1980.

Lippman, M. E., Yarbro, G. K., and Leventhal, B. G. "Effects of Glucocorticoids on F_c Receptors of a Human Granulocyte Cell Line." *Cancer Research*, 1978, *38*, 4251-4256.

Lo, B., and Jonsen, A. "Ethical Decisions in the Care of a Patient Terminally Ill with Metastatic Cancer." *Annals of Internal Medicine*, 1980, *92*, 107–111.

Loosen, O., and Prange, A. "Serum Thyrotropin Response to TRH in Psychiatric Patients: A Review." *American Journal of Psychiatry*, 1982, *139*, 405–416.

Luparello, T. J., Stein, M., and Park, C. D. "Effect of Hypothalamic Lesions on Rat Anaphylaxis." *American Journal of Physiology*, 1964, *207*, 911–914.

Lyon, J., Gardner, J., and West, D. "Cancer Incidence in Mormons and Non-Mormons in Utah During 1967–75." *Journal of the National Cancer Institute*, 1980, *65*, 1055–1061.

McCusker, J., and Morrow, G. "Factors Related to the Use of Cancer Early Detection Techniques." *Preventive Medicine*, 1980, *9*, 388–397.

McCusker, J., Wax, A., and Bennett, J. "Cancer Patient Accessions into Clinical Trials." *American Journal of Clinical Oncology*, 1982, *5*, 227–236.

McGuire, W. L. "An Update on Estrogen and Progesterone Receptors in Prognosis for Primary and Advanced Breast Cancer." In S. Iacobelli (ed.), *Hormones and Cancer*. New York: Raven Press, 1980.

Mack, T., Pike, M., and Henderson, B. "Estrogens and Endometrial Cancer in a Retirement Community." *New England Journal of Medicine*, 1976, *294*, 1262–1267.

Maclean, D., and Reichlin, S. "Neuroendocrinology and the Immune Process." In R. Ader (ed.), *Psychoneuroimmunology*. Orlando, Fla.: Academic Press, 1981.

Maclure, K., and MacMahon, B. "An Epidemiological Perspective of Environmental Carcinogenesis." *Epidemiology Review*, 1980, *2*, 19–48.

McNeil, B., and Eddy, D. "The Costs and Effects of Screening for Cancer Among Asbestos-Exposed Workers." *Journal of Chronic Diseases*, 1982, *35*, 351–358.

Macris, N. T., Schiavi, R. C., Camerino, M. S., and Stein, M. "Effect of Hypothalamic Lesions on Immune Processes in the Guinea Pig." *American Journal of Physiology*, 1970, *219*, 1205–1209.

Magnus, K. "Incidence of Malignant Melanoma of the Skin in the Five Nordic Countries: Significance of Solar Radiation." *International Journal of Cancer*, 1977, *20*, 477–485.

Manfredi, C., Warneke, R., Graham, S., and Rosenthal, S. "Social Psychological Correlates of Health Behavior: Knowledge of Breast Self-Examination Techniques Among Black Women." *Social Science and Medicine*, 1977, *11*, 433–440.

Marsh, J. T., and Rasmussen, A. F. "Response of Adrenal, Thymus, Spleen, and Leukocytes to Shuttle Box and Confinement Stress." *Proceedings of the Society for Experimental Biology and Medicine*, 1960, *104*, 180–183.

Marx, J. "The N-myc Oncogene in Neural Tumors." *Science*, 1984a, *224*, 1088.

Marx, J. "Oncogenes Amplified in Cancer Cells." *Science*, 1984b, *223*, 40–41.

Marx, J. "AIDS Virus Genomes." *Science*, 1985, *227*, 503.

Mashberg, A., Garfinkel, L., and Harris, S. "Alcohol as a Primary Risk Factor in Oral Squamous Carcinoma." *Ca-A Cancer Journal for Clinicians*, 1981, *31*, 146–155.

Mason, J. W. "Psychologic Stress and Endocrine Function." In E. J. Sachar (ed.), *Topics in Psychoendocrinology*. Orlando, Fla.: Grune & Stratton, 1975.

Mason, J. W., and others. "Concurrent Plasma Epinephrine, Norepinephrine, and 17-Hydroxycorticosteroid Levels During Conditioned Emotional Disturbances in Monkeys." *Psychosomatic Medicine*, 1961, *23*, 344–348.

Mathe, A. A., Yen, S. S., Sohn, R. J., and Kemper, T. "Effect of Hypothalamic Lesions on Anaphylactic Release of PSs from Guinea Pig Lung." Paper presented at 7th International Congress on Pharmacology, Paris, 1978.

Mathews, P., Froelich, D., Sibbitt, W., and Bankhurst, A. "Enhancement of Natural Cytotoxicity by B-Endorphin." *Journal of Immunology*, 1983, *130*, 1658–1662.

Mausner, B., Mausner, J., and Rial, W. "The Influence of a Physician on the Smoking Behavior of His Patients." In S. Zagna (ed.), *Studies and Issues in Smoking Behavior*. Tucson: University of Arizona Press, 1967.

Mausner, J. "Cigarette Smoking Among Patients with Respiratory Disease." *American Review of Respiratory Disease*, 1970, *102*, 704–713.

Mendelsohn, J., Multer, M. M., and Bernheim, J. L. "Inhibition of Human Lymphocyte Stimulation by Steroid Hormones: Cytokinetic Mechanisms." *Clinical and Experimental Immunology*, 1977, *27*, 127–134.

Merleau-Ponty, M. *Phenomenology of Perception*. London: Routledge & Kegan Paul, 1962.

Mettlin, C. "Nutritional Habits of Blacks and Whites." *Preventive Medicine*, 1980, *9*, 601–606.

Mettlin, C., and Murphy, G. *Issues in Cancer Screening and Communications*. New York: Alan R. Liss, 1982.

Michaut, R. J., and others. "Influence of Early Maternal Deprivation on Adult Humoral Immune Reponse in Mice." *Physiology and Behavior*, 1981, *26*, 189–191.

Miczek, K., and Thompson, M. "Analgesia Resulting from Defeat in a Social Confrontation: The Role of Endogenous Opioids in Brain." In R. Bandler (ed.), *Modulation of Sensorimotor Activity During Altered Behavioral States*. New York: Alan R. Liss, 1984.

Milham, S. *Occupational Mortality in Washington State, 1950–1971*. DHEW No. NIOSH-76-175. Washington, D.C.: U.S. Government Printing Office, 1976.

Miller, A. "Evaluation of Screening for Cancer of the Cervix and Breast: Implications for Cancer Control." In C. Mettlin and G. Murphy (eds.), *Issues in Cancer Screening and Communications*. New York: Alan R. Liss, 1982.

Miller, G., Murgo, A., and Plotnikoff, N. "Enkephalins— Enhancement of Active T-Cell Rosettes from Normal Volunteers." *Clinical Immunology and Immunopathology*, 1984, *31*, 132–137.

Miller, J. *Living Systems*. New York: McGraw-Hill, 1978.

Miller, M. "Decision-Making in the Death Process of the Ill Aged." *Geriatrics*, 1971, *26*, 105–116.

Miller, P. "Principles of Early Detection of Cancer." *Cancer*, 1981, *47*, 1142–1145.

Miller, T., and Spratt, J. S. "Critical Review of Reported Psychological Correlates of Cancer Prognosis and Growth."

In B. A. Stoll (ed.), *Mind and Cancer Prognosis*. New York: Wiley, 1979.

Mills, J. E., and Widdicomb, J. G. "Role of the Vagus Verves in Anaphylaxis and Histamine-Induced Bronchoconstriction in Guinea Pigs." *British Journal of Pharmacology*, 1970, *39*, 724-731.

Moertel, C., and others. "A Clinical Trial of Amygdalin (Laetrile) in the Treatment of Human Cancer." *New England Journal of Medicine*, 1982, *306*, 201-206.

Monjan, A. A., and Collector, M. I. "Stress-Induced Modulation of the Immune Response." *Science*, 1977, *196*, 307-308.

Moody, T. W., and others. "High Levels of Intracellular Bombesin Characterize Human Small-Cell Lung Carcinoma." *Science*, 1981, *214*, 1246-1250.

Moore, O., and Foote, F. "The Relatively Favorable Prognosis of Medullary Carcinoma." *Cancer*, 1949, *2*, 635-642.

Morrow, G., Way, J., Hoagland, A., and Cooper, R. "Patient Compliance with Self-Directed Hemoccult Testing." *Preventive Medicine*, 1982, *11*, 512-520.

Mulvihill, J., Safyer, A., and Bening, J. "Prevention in Familial Breast Cancer: Counseling and Prophylactic Mastectomy." *Preventive Medicine*, 1982, *11*, 500-511.

Mushinski, M., and Stellman, S. D. "Impact of New Smoking Trends on Women's Occupational Health." *Preventive Medicine*, 1978, *7*, 349-365.

Nagy, E., and Berczi, I. "Immunodeficiency in Hypophysectomized Rats." *Acta Endocrinologica*, 1978, *89*, 530-537.

Nahmias, A., Naib, Z., and Highsmith, A. "Experimental Genital Herpes Simplex Infection in the Mouse." *Pediatrics Research*, 1967, *1*, 209.

Nahmias, A., Naib, Z., and Josey, W. "Prospective Studies of the Association of Genital Herpes Simplex Infection and Cervical Anaplasia." *Cancer Research*, 1973, *33*, 1491-1497.

Nathanson, L. "Immunology and Immunotherapy of Human Breast Cancer." *Cancer Immunology and Immunotherapy*, 1977, *7*, 209-224.

National Center for Health Statistics. "Characterization of Females Having a Pap Smear and Interval Since Last Pap

Smear.'' *United States Monthly Vital Statistics Report*, 1975, *24* (supp.), 1-8.

National Institute for Occupational Safety and Health. *Special Occupational Hazard Review of Trichloroethylene*. DHEW Publication No. 78-130. Washington, D.C.: U.S. Government Printing Office, 1978.

Nilzen, A. "The Influence of the Thyroid Gland on Hypersensitivity Reactions in Animals." *Acta Allergologica*, 1955, *7*, 231-234.

Nitschke, R., and others. "Therapeutic Choices Made by Patients with End-Stage Cancer." *Behavioral Pediatrics*, 1982, *101*, 471-476.

Pack, G., and Gallo, J. "Culpability for Delay in Treatment of Cancer." *American Journal of Cancer*, 1938, *33*, 443-462.

Palmblad, J., and others. "Lymphocyte and Granulocyte Reactions During Sleep Deprivation." *Psychosomatic Medicine*, 1979, *41*, 273-278.

Parker, C. W. "Adrenergic Responsiveness in Asthma." In K. F. Austen and L. M. Lichtenstein (eds.), *Asthma Physiology, Immunopharmacology, and Treatment*. Orlando, Fla.: Academic Press, 1973.

Pater, J., Loeb, M., and Siu, T. "A Multivariate Analysis of the Contribution of 'Auxometry' to Prognosis in Breast Cancer." *Journal of Chronic Diseases*, 1979, *32*, 375-384.

Pederson, L. "Compliance with Physician Advice to Quit Smoking: A Review of the Literature." *Preventive Medicine*, 1982, *11*, 71-84.

Pederson, L., Williams, J., and Lefcoe, N. "Smoking Cessation Among Pulmonary Patients as Related to Type of Respiratory Disease and Demographic Variables." *Canadian Journal of Public Health*, 1980, *71*, 191-194.

Pendergrass, T., and Davis, S. "Knowledge and Use of 'Alternative' Cancer Therapies in Children." *American Journal of Pediatric Hematology/Oncology*, 1981, *3*, 339-345.

Peterson, C., Seligman, M., and Luborsky, L. "Attributions and Depressive Mood Shifts: A Case Study Using the Symptom-Context Method." *Journal of Abnormal Psychology*, 1983, *92*, 96-103.

Petrovski, I. N. "Problems of Nervous Control in Immunity Reactions." *Mikrobiologica Epidemiologica Immunobiologica*, 1961, *32*, 63–69.

Pettingale, K. W., Greer, S., and Tee, D. E. "Serum IgA and Emotional Expression in Breast Cancer Patients." *Journal of Psychosomatic Research*, 1977, *21*, 395–399.

Pierce, G., Shikes, R., and Fink, L. *Cancer: A Problem of Developmental Biology.* Englewood Cliffs, N.J.: Prentice-Hall, 1978.

Pochet, R., Delesperse, G., Gauseet, P. W., and Collet, H. "Distribution of Beta-Adrenergic Receptors on Human Lymphocyte Subpopulations." *Clinical and Experimental Immunology*, 1979, *38*, 578–584.

Poh-Fitzpatrick, M. "The Biologic Actions of Solar Radiation on Skin, with a Note on Sunscreens." *Journal of Dermatology*, 1977, *3*, 199–204.

Polanyi, M. *The Study of Man.* Chicago: University of Chicago Press, 1958.

Popovic, M., Sarngadharan, M., Read, E., and Gallo, R. "Detection, Isolation, and Continuous Production of Cytopathic Retroviruses (HTLV-III) from Patients with AIDS and pre-AIDS." *Science*, 1984, *224*, 497–500.

Pottern, L., and others. "Esophageal Cancer Among Black Men in Washington D.C. I: Alcohol, Tobacco, and Other Risk Factors." *Journal of the National Cancer Institute*, 1981, *67*, 777–783.

Pross, H., and Baines, M. "Spontaneous Human Lymphocyte-Mediated Cytotoxicity Against Tumour Target Cells. I: The Effect of Malignant Disease." *International Journal of Cancer*, 1976, *18*, 593–604.

Rawls, W., and others. "Genital Herpes in Two Social Groups." *American Journal of Obstetrics and Gynecology*, 1971, *110*, 682–689.

Repcekova, D., and Mikulaj, L. "Plasma Testosterone of Rats Subjected to Immobilization Stress and/or HCG Administration." *Hormone Research*, 1977, *8*, 51–55.

Rice, R. W., Abe, K., and Critchlow, V. "Abolition of Plasma Growth Hormone Response to Stress and of the Circadian Rhythm in Pituitary-Adrenal Function in Female Rats with

Preoptic-Anterior Hypothalamic Lesions." *Brain Research*, 1978, *148*, 129–141.

Richardson, A., and Lyon, J. "The Effect of Condom Use on Squamous Cell Cervical Intraepithelial Neoplasia." *American Journal of Obstetrics and Gynecology*, 1981, *140*, 909–913.

Riley, V. "Psychoneuroendocrine Influences on Immunocompetence and Neoplasia." *Science*, 1981, *212*, 1100–1109.

Riley, V., Fitzmaurice, M., and Spackman, D. "Immuno-Competence and Neoplasia: Role of Anxiety Stress." In S. Levy (ed.), *Biological Mediators of Behavior and Disease: Neoplasia*. New York: Elsevier Science, 1982.

Rogentine, N., and others. "Psychological Factors in the Prognosis of Malignant Melanoma: A Prospective Study." *Psychosomatic Medicine*, 1979, *41*, 647–655.

Rogot, E., and Murray, J. "Smoking and Causes of Death Among U.S. Veterans: 16 Years of Observation." *Public Health Reports*, 1980, *95*, 213–222.

Room, R. "Measurements of Drinking Patterns in the General Population and Possible Applications in Studies of the Role of Alcohol in Cancer." *Cancer Research*, 1979, *39*, 2830–2833.

Rose, R. M., and Sacher, E. "Psychoendocrinology." In R. H. Williams (ed.), *Textbook of Endocrinology*. Philadelphia: Saunders, 1981.

Rothman, K., and Keller, R. "The Effect of Joint Exposure to Alcohol and Tobacco on Risk of Cancer of the Mouth and Pharynx." *Journal of Chronic Diseases*, 1972, *25*, 711–716.

Rubin, P., and Bennett, J. "Ovarian Cancer." In P. Rubin (ed.), *Clinical Oncology for Medical Students and Physicians*. New York: American Cancer Society, 1978.

Russell, M., and Welte, J. "Drinking Patterns of U.S. Women from the Health and Nutrition Examination Surveys, 1971–1973." Paper presented at 26th annual forum of the National Council on Alcoholism, Washington, D.C., Apr. 27, 1979.

Russell, M., Wilson, C., Taylor, C., and Baker, C. "Effect of General Practitioners' Advice Against Smoking." *British Medical Journal*, 1979, *2*, 231–235.

Sacher, E., and Baron, M. "The Biology of Affective Disorders." *Annual Review of Neurosciences*, 1979, *2*, 505–517.

Salazar, O. "Endometrium." In P. Rubin (ed.), *Clinical Oncology for Medical Students and Physicians*. New York: American Cancer Society, 1978.

Sato, G. "Towards an Endocrine Physiology of Human Cancer." In S. Iacobelli (ed.), *Hormones and Cancer*. New York: Raven Press, 1980.

Schiavi, R. C., Adams, J., and Stein, M. "Effect of Hypothalamic Lesions on Histamine Toxicity in the Guinea Pig." *American Journal of Physiology*, 1966, *211*, 1269–1273.

Schiavi, R. C., Macris, N. T., Camerino, M. S., and Stein, M. "Effect of Hypothalamic Lesions on Immediate Hypersensitivity." *American Journal of Physiology*, 1975, *228*, 596–601.

Schleifer, S. J., and others. "Suppression of Lymphocyte Stimulation Following Bereavement." *Journal of the American Medical Association*, 1983, *250*, 374–377.

Schleifer, S. J., and others. "Depression and Immunity." *Archives of General Psychiatry*, 1984, *42*, 129–133.

Schottenfeld, D. "Alcohol as a Co-Factor in the Etiology of Cancer." *Cancer*, 1979, *43*, 1962–1966.

Schupbach, J., and others. "Serological Analysis of a Subgroup of Human T-Lymphotropic Retroviruses (HTLV-III) Associated with AIDS." *Science*, 1984, *224*, 503–505.

Schutz, A. *Collected Papers*. Vol. 1: *The Problem of Social Reality*. (M. Nathanson, ed.) The Hague: Nijhoff, 1973.

Schwartz, G. "Disregulation Theory and Disease: Applications to the Repression/Cerebral Disconnection/Cardiovascular Disorder Hypothesis." *International Review of Applied Psychology*, 1983, *32*, 95–118.

Schwoon, D., and Schmoll, H. J. "Motivation to Participate in Cancer Screening Programs." *Social Science and Medicine*, 1979, *13A*, 283–286.

Seligman, M., and Beagley, G. "Learned Helplessness in the Rat." *Journal of Comparative and Physiological Psychology*, 1975, *88*, 534–541.

Selikoff, I., Hammond, E., and Churg, J. "Asbestos Exposure, Smoking, and Neoplasia." *Journal of the American Medical Association*, 1968, *204*, 104–110.

Shapiro, S. "Evidence on Screening for Breast Cancer from a Randomized Trial." *Cancer*, 1977, *39*, 2772-2782.

Shavit, J., and others. "Opioid Peptides Mediate the Suppressive Effect of Stress on Natural Killer Cell Cytotoxicity." *Science*, 1984, *223*, 188-190.

Shekelle, R. B., and others. "Psychological Depression and 17 Year Risk of Death from Cancer." *Psychosomatic Medicine*, 1981, *43*, 117-125.

Sherin, K. "Smoking Cessation: The Physician's Role." *Postgraduate Medicine*, 1982, *72*, 99-106.

Shimokawara, I., and others. "Identification of Lymphocyte Subpopulations in Human Breast Cancer Tissue and Its Significance." *Cancer*, 1982, *49*, 1456-1464.

Sillett, R., Wilson, M., and Malcolm, R. "Deception Among Smokers." *British Medical Journal*, 1978, *2*, 1185-1186.

Skegg, D., Corwin, P., Paul, C., and Doll, R. "Importance of the Male Factor in Cancer of the Cervix." *Lancet*, 1982, *2*, 581-583.

Sklar, L., and Anisman, H. "Stress and Coping Factors Influence Tumor Growth." *Science*, 1979, *205*, 513-515.

Sklar, L., and Anisman, H. "Stress and Cancer." *Psychological Bulletin*, 1981, *89*, 369-406.

Smith, E. "Epidemiology of Oral and Pharyngeal Cancers in the United States: Review of Recent Literature." *Journal of the National Cancer Institute*, 1979, *63*, 1189-1198.

Smith, H. "Myocardial Infarction—Case Studies of Ethics in the Consent Situation." *Social Science and Medicine*, 1974, *8*, 399-404.

Smith, S., Cairns, N., Sturgeon, J., and Lansky, S. "Poor Drug Compliance in an Adolescent with Leukemia." *American Journal of Pediatric Hematology/Oncology*, 1981, *3*, 297-300.

Smith, S., Rosen, D., Trueworthy, R., and Lowman, J. "A Reliable Method for Evaluating Drug Compliance in Children with Cancer." *Cancer*, 1979, *43*, 169-173.

Sobel, H. *Behavioral Thanatology*. Cambridge, Mass.: Ballinger, 1981.

Solomon, G. F. "Stress and Antibody Response in Rats." *International Archives of Allergy*, 1969, *35*, 97-104.

Sonnabend, J., Witkin, S., and Purtilo, D. "Acquired Immune

Deficiency Syndrome, Opportunistic Infections, and Malignancies in Male Homosexuals: A Hypothesis of Etiologic Factors in Pathogenesis." *Journal of the American Medical Association*, 1983, *249*, 2370–2374.

Sontag, S. *Illness as Metaphor*. New York: Farrar, Straus & Giroux, 1978.

Spitzer, R. L., Endicott, J., and Robins, E. "Research Diagnostic Criteria: Rationale and Reliability." *Archives of General Psychiatry*, 1978, *35*, 773–782.

Stahl, R., and others. "Immunologic Abnormalities in Homosexual Men: Relationship to Kaposi's Sarcoma." *American Journal of Medicine*, 1982, *73*, 171–178.

Steinhauer, E., Doyle, A., Reed, J., and Kadish, A. "Defective Natural Cytotoxicity in Patients with Cancer: Normal Number of Effector Cells but Decreased Recycling Capacity in Patients with Advanced Disease." *Journal of Immunology*, 1982, *129*, 2255–2259.

Stellman, S., and Stellman, J. "Women's Occupations, Smoking, and Cancer and Other Diseases." *Ca-A Cancer Journal for Clinicians*, 1981, *31*, 29–42.

Sterling, T. "Does Smoking Kill Workers or Working Kill Smokers? Or the Mutual Relationship Between Smoking, Occupation, and Respiratory Disease." *International Journal of Health Services*, 1978, *8*, 437–452.

Stoll, B. *Mind and Cancer Prognosis*. New York: Wiley, 1979.

Stoll, B. (ed.). *Prolonged Arrest of Cancer*. New York: Wiley, 1982.

Szentivanyi, A., and Szekely, J. "Anaphylaxis and the Nervous System. Part II." *Annals of Allergy*, 1958, *16*, 389–392.

Tamarkin, L., and others. "Decreased Nocturnal Plasma Melatonin Peak in Patients with Estrogen Receptor Positive Breast Cancer." *Science*, 1982, *216*, 1003–1005.

Tannenbaum, A. "The Genesis and Growth of Tumors. II: Effects of Caloric Restriction per se." *Cancer Research*, 1942, *3*, 460–467.

Taylor, K., Margolese, R., and Soskolne, C. "Physicians' Reasons for Not Entering Eligible Patients in a Randomized Clinical Trial of Surgery for Breast Cancer." *New England Journal of Medicine*, 1984, *316*, 1363–1367.

Thanavala, Y. M., Rao, S. S., and Thakur, A. N. "The Effect of an Aestrogenic Steroid on the Secondary Immune Response Under Different Hormonal Environments." *Acta Endocrinologica*, 1973, *72*, 582–586.

Thomas, C. (ed.). *The Precursors Study: A Prospective Study of a Cohort of Medical Students*. Vol. 5. Baltimore: Johns Hopkins University Press, 1983.

Thomson, S. P., McMahon, L. J., and Nugent, C. A. "Endogenous Cortisol: A Regulator of the Number of Lymphocytes in Peripheral Blood." *Clinical Immunology and Immunopathology*, 1980, *17*, 506–514.

Thrasher, S. G., Bernardis, L. L., and Cohen, S. "The Immune Response in Hypothalamic-Lesioned and Hypophysectomized Rats." *International Archives of Allergy*, 1971, *41*, 813–820.

Tolstoy, L. *"The Death of Ivan Ilych" and Other Stories*. (Originally published 1886.) (M. Aylmer, trans.) New York: New American Library, 1960.

Trichopoulos, D., Kalandidi, A., Sparros, L., and MacMahon, B. "Lung Cancer and Passive Smoking." *International Journal of Cancer*, 1981, *27*, 1–4.

Tyrey, L., and Nalbandov, A. V. "Influence of Anterior Hypothalamic Lesions on Circulating Antibody Titers in the Rat." *American Journal of Physiology*, 1972, *222*, 179–185.

Vessey, S. H. "Effects of Grouping on Levels of Circulating Antibodies in Mice." *Proceedings of the Society for Biology*, 1964, *115*, 252–255.

Visintainer, M. A., and Casey, R. "Adjustment and Outcome in Melanoma Patients." Paper presented at meeting of the American Psychological Association, Toronto, 1984.

Visintainer, M. A., Volpicelli, J. R., and Seligman, M. E. P. "Tumor Rejection in Rats After Inescapable or Escapable Shock." *Science*, 1982, *216*, 437–439.

Wainwright, J. "The Reduction of Cancer Mortality." *New England Journal of Medicine*, 1911, *95*, 1165–1168.

Watson, A. "Artificial Tanning and Suntan Salons." *Medical Journal of Australia*, 1982, *1*, 430–431.

Weber, R., and Pert, C. "Opiatergic Modulation of the Immune System." In E. Müller and A. Genazzani (eds.), *Cen-*

tral and Peripheral Endorphins: Basic and Clinical Aspects. New York: Raven Press, 1984.

Weiss, J., Glazer, H., Pohorecky, L., and Miller, N. "Effects of Chronic Exposure to Stressors on Avoidance-Escape Behavior and on Brain Norepinephrine." *Psychosomatic Medicine,* 1975, *37,* 522–534.

West, D., Lyon, J., and Gardner, J. "Cancer Risk Factors: An Analysis of Utah Mormons and Non-Mormons." *Journal of the National Cancer Institute,* 1980, *65,* 1083–1095.

Wheelock, E., and Robinson, M. "Endogenous Control of the Neoplastic Process." *Laboratory Investigation,* 1983, *48,* 120–139.

Wheelock, E., Weinhold, K., and Levich, J. "The Tumor Dormant State." *Advances in Cancer Research,* 1981, *34,* 107–140.

Whittier, J. R., and Orr, A. "Hyperkinesia and Other Physiologic Effects of Caudate Deficit in the Adult Albino Rat." *Neurology,* 1962, *12,* 529–539.

Whybrow, R., and Prange, A. "A Hypothesis of Thyroid Catecholamine Receptor Interaction." *Archives of General Psychiatry,* 1981, *38,* 106–113.

Wilkinson, G., and others. "Delay, Stage of Disease and Survival from Breast Cancer." *Journal of Chronic Diseases,* 1979, *32,* 365–373.

Williams, J. W., and others. "Sympathetic Innervation of Murine Thymus and Spleen: Evidence for a Functional Link Between the Nervous and Immune Systems." *Brain Research Bulletin,* 1980, *6,* 83–94.

Winawer, S. "Screening for Colorectal Cancer: An Overview." *Cancer,* 1980, *45,* 1093–1098.

Winn, D., and others. "Snuff Dipping and Oral Cancer Among Women in the Southern United States." *New England Journal of Medicine,* 1981, *304,* 745–749.

Worden, W., and Weisman, A. "Psychosocial Components of Lagtime in Cancer Diagnosis." *Journal of Psychosomatic Research,* 1975, *19,* 69–79.

World Health Organization, Scientific Group on Prevention Strategies in Cancer. *Draft Report.* Geneva: World Health Organization, 1981.

Wright, N., and Riopelle, M. "Age at Time of First Intercourse v. Chronologic Age as a Basis for Pap Smear Screening." *Canadian Medical Association Journal*, 1982, *127*, 126–131.

Wright, N., and others. "Neoplasia and Dysplasia of the Cervix Uteri and Contraception: A Possible Protective Effect of the Diaphragm." *British Journal of Cancer*, 1978, *38*, 273–279.

Wyle, F. A., and Kent, J. R. "Immunosuppression by Sex Steroid Hormones." *Clinical and Experimental Immunology*, 1977, *27*, 407–415.

Yu, S., Miller, A., and Sherman, G. "Optimizing the Age, Number of Tests and Test Interval for Cervical Screening in Canada." *Journal of Epidemiology and Community Health*, 1981, *36*, 1–10.

Yuhus, J., and Tarleton, A. "Dormancy and Spontaneous Recurrence of Human Breast Cancer *in vitro*." *Cancer Research*, 1978, *38*, 3584–3589.

Zagon, I., and McLaughlin, P. "Naloxone Prolongs the Survival Time of Mice Treated with Neuroblastoma." *Life Sciences*, 1981, *28*, 1095–1102.

Ziegler, R., and others. "Esophageal Cancer Among Black Men in Washington, D.C. II: Role of Nutrition." *Journal of the National Cancer Institute*, 1981, *67*, 1199–1206.

Name Index

Subject Index